POCKET REFERENCE TO

The

12-Lead ECG
in Acute Coronary
Syndromes

POCKET REFERENCE TO

The

12-LEAD ECG
IN ACUTE CORONARY
SYNDROMES

TIM PHALEN

BARBARA AEHLERT

SECOND EDITION

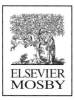

ELSEVIER
MOSBY

ELSEVIER
MOSBY

11830 Westline Industrial Drive
St. Louis, Missouri 63146

POCKET REFERENCE TO   ISBN 0-323-03762-3
THE 12-LEAD ECG IN ACUTE CORONARY
SYNDROMES
Copyright © 2006 by Mosby, Inc.

NOTICE

Pharmacology is an ever-changing field. Standard safety precautions must be
followed, but as new research and clinical experience broaden our
knowledge, changes in treatment and drug therapy may become necessary or
appropriate. Readers are advised to check the most current product
information provided by the manufacturer of each drug to be administered to
verify the recommended dose, the method and duration of administration,
and contraindications. It is the responsibility of the licensed prescriber,
relying on experience and knowledge of the patient, to determine dosages
and the best treatment for each individual patient. Neither the publisher nor
the editor assumes any liability for any injury and/or damage to persons or
property arising from this publication.

International Standard Book Number 0-323-03762-3

Publishing Director: Andrew Allen
Acquisitions Editor: Linda Honeycutt
Associate Developmental Editor: Katherine Tomber
Publishing Services Manager: Julie Eddy
Designer: Jyotika Shroff

Printed in China

Last digit is the print number: 9   8   7   6   5   4   3   2   1

To my Dad
James T. Phalen

ACKNOWLEDGMENTS

We would like to thank the people that have been helpful to us in the completion of this project.

- We would like to thank Linda Honeycutt and the Elsevier editorial team for their extraordinary work on this project. Thank you for providing us with an occasional nudge and the necessary resources to complete this book.

Tim Phalen
Barbara Aehlert

Contents

1   Reviewing the Basics, 1

2   Introduction to the 12-Lead ECG, 14

3   Acquiring the 12-lead ECG, 36

4   Acute Coronary Syndromes, 49

5   Myocardial Infarction: Recognition and Localization, 71

6   Myocardial Infarction: Complications and Treatment, 103

7   Bundle Branch Block, 118

8   Acute Coronary Syndromes Imitators, 131

References, 146

Ilustration Credits, 147

Index, 150

POCKET REFERENCE TO

The

12-Lead ECG
in Acute Coronary
Syndromes

CHAPTER 1

Reviewing the Basics

Location of the Heart

The heart is a hollow muscular organ that lies in the middle of the thoracic cavity (mediastinum) behind the sternum, between the lungs, and just above the diaphragm. It is surrounded by a protective sac (pericardium) and is attached to the thorax through the great vessels (pulmonary arteries and veins, aorta, superior and inferior vena cavae) (Figure 1-1).

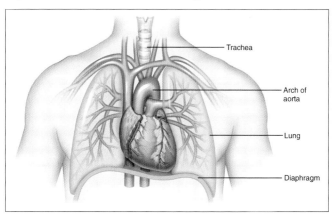

Trachea

Arch of aorta

Lung

Diaphragm

FIGURE **1-1** Location of the heart. The heart lies in the middle of the thoracic cavity (mediastinum) behind the sternum and between the lungs.

The apex of the heart is formed by the tip of the left ventricle. It is positioned just above the diaphragm to the left in an anterior position at the fifth intercostal space, midclavicular line. The base (top) of the heart is at approximately the level of the second intercostal space. The anterior surface of the heart consists primarily of the right ventricle.

Heart Chambers

The heart is divided into four cavities, or chambers, but functions as a two-sided pump. The two upper chambers are the right and left atria, and the two lower chambers are the right and left ventricles. The right side of the heart is a low-pressure system that pumps venous blood to the lungs. The left side is a high-pressure system that pumps arterial blood to the systemic circulation.

The *atria* are thin walled, low-pressure chambers that receive blood. An internal wall of connective tissue called the *interatrial septum* separates the right and left atria. The right atrium receives deoxygenated blood from the superior vena cava (which carries blood from the head and upper extremities), the inferior vena cava (which carries blood from the lower body), and the coronary sinus (which receives blood from the intracardiac circulation). The left atrium receives oxygenated blood from the lungs via the right and left pulmonary veins.

The *ventricles* pump blood to the lungs and systemic circulation. An internal wall of connective tissue called the *interventricular septum* separates the right and left ventricles. The ventricles are larger and have thicker walls than the atria. The left ventricle is a high-pressure chamber that is about three times thicker than the right ventricle. To pump blood out of the left ventricle to the systemic circulation, the left ventricle must contract forcefully and overcome arterial pressure and resistance. Each ventricle holds about 150 mL when full and normally ejects only about half this volume (70 to 80 mL) with each contraction.

Layers of the Heart

The heart wall is made up of three tissue layers: the endocardium, myocardium, and epicardium. The *endocardium* (innermost layer) is a thin, smooth layer of epithelium and connective tissue that lines the heart's inner chambers, valves, chordae tendineae, and papillary muscles. The endocardium is continuous with the innermost layer *(tunica intima)* of the arteries, veins, and capillaries of the body, creating a continuous, closed circulatory system.

The *myocardium* (middle layer) is a thick, muscular layer that consists of cardiac muscle fibers (cells) responsible for the pumping action of the heart. The myocardium is subdivided into two areas. The innermost half of the myocardium is called the *subendocardial area* and the outermost half is called the *subepicardial area.* The muscle fibers of the myocardium are separated by connective tissues that are richly supplied with capillaries and nerve fibers.

The *epicardium* is the external layer of the heart, and it includes blood capillaries, lymph capillaries, nerve fibers, and fat. The main coronary arteries cross this layer before entering the myocardium. The *pericardium* is a double walled sac that encloses the heart and helps protect it from trauma and infection.

Valves of the Heart

The heart has four valves: two sets of atrioventricular (AV) valves and two sets of semilunar valves (Table 1-1). Their purpose is to ensure blood flow in one direction through the heart's chambers and prevent the backflow of blood.

TABLE **1-1**	**Heart Valves**	
Valve type	**Name**	**Location**
Atrioventricular	Tricuspid	Separates right atrium and right ventricle
	Mitral (bicuspid)	Separates left atrium and left ventricle
Semilunar	Pulmonic	Between right ventricle and pulmonary artery
	Aortic	Between left ventricle and aorta

The AV valves separate the atria from the ventricles. The tricuspid valve lies between the right atrium and right ventricle. It consists of three separate leaflets. The mitral (or bicuspid) valve has only two cusps and lies between the left atrium and left ventricle.

The pulmonic and aortic valves are semilunar (SL) valves that prevent backflow of blood from the aorta and pulmonary arteries into the ventricles during diastole. Both sets of SL valves have three cusps shaped like half-moons.

Blood Flow Through the Heart

The right atrium receives blood low in oxygen and high in carbon dioxide from the superior and inferior vena cavae and the coronary sinus (Figure 1-2). Blood flows from the right atrium through the tricuspid valve into the right ventricle. When the right ventricle contracts, the tricuspid valve closes. The right ventricle expels the blood through the pulmonic valve into the pulmonary trunk. The pulmonary trunk divides into a right and left pulmonary artery, each of which carries blood to one lung (pulmonary circuit).

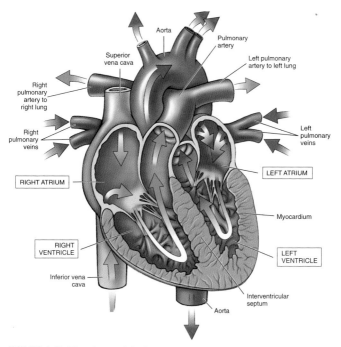

FIGURE **1-2** Chambers of the heart and the large vessels. Arrows show the flow of blood through the heart.

Blood flows through the pulmonary arteries to the lungs (where oxygen and carbon dioxide are exchanged in the pulmonary capillaries) and then to the pulmonary veins. Carbon dioxide is exhaled as the left atrium receives oxygenated blood from the lungs via the four pulmonary veins (two from the right lung and two from the left lung). Blood flows from the left atrium through the mitral (bicuspid) valve into the left ventricle. When the left ventricle contracts, the mitral valve closes. Blood leaves the left ventricle through the aortic valve to the aorta and its branches and is distributed throughout the body *(systemic circuit).* Blood from the tissues of the head, neck, and upper extremities is emptied into the superior vena cava. Blood from the lower body is emptied into the inferior vena cava. The superior and inferior vena cavae carry their contents into the right atrium.

Coronary Circulation

The coronary circulation consists of coronary arteries and veins. With normal activity, 65% to 75% of the arterial oxygen content in the blood is extracted by the myocardium through the coronary arteries. Myocardial ischemia results when the heart's demand for oxygen exceeds its supply from the coronary circulation.

Blood is supplied to the tissues of the heart during diastole by the first two branches of the aorta: the right and left coronary arteries (Figure 1-3). The openings to these vessels are just beyond the cusps of the aortic SL valve. The coronary arteries cross the epicardium and branch several times. These branches enter the myocardium and endocardium and further divide to become arterioles and then capillaries. The coronary arteries receive their blood supply during diastole or when the ventricular muscle mass is relaxing.

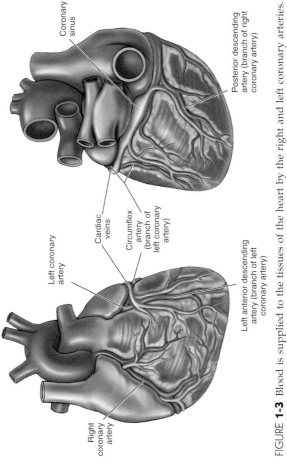

FIGURE 1-3 Blood is supplied to the tissues of the heart by the right and left coronary arteries. The left coronary artery branches into the left anterior descending artery and the circumflex artery. The coronary veins collect blood and empty it into the coronary sinus, which eventually empties into the right atrium.

Right Coronary Artery

The right coronary artery (RCA) originates from the right side of the aorta and passes along the AV sulcus between the right atrium and right ventricle. The marginal branch of the RCA supplies the right atrium and right ventricle. In 50% to 60% of individuals, a branch of the RCA supplies the sinoatrial (SA) node. In 85% to 90% of hearts, the RCA also branches into the AV node artery.

The posterior descending artery supplies blood to the walls of both ventricles. This vessel has several branches including the septal branch that supplies the posterior third of the interventricular septum.

Left Coronary Artery

The left coronary artery (LCA) originates from the left side of the aorta. The first segment of the LCA is called the *left main coronary artery.* It is approximately the width of a soda straw and less than an inch long. The left main coronary artery divides into two primary branches: the *left anterior descending* (LAD) (also called the *anterior interventricular*) artery and the *left circumflex* (LCx) artery. These vessels are slightly smaller than the left main coronary artery. Branches of the LAD, the diagonal and septal arteries, supply blood to the anterior surfaces of both ventricles. The LAD is embedded in the epicardial surface of the anterior surface of the heart.

The left circumflex coronary artery circles around the left side of the heart and is embedded in the epicardium on the back of the heart. The LCx branch supplies blood to the left atrium and the lateral wall of the left ventricle. In some patients, the circumflex artery may also supply the inferior portion of the left ventricle. If the posterior wall of the left ventricle is damaged, a cardiac catheterization is usually necessary to determine which coronary artery is involved because both the RCA and LCx supply blood to this area.

Coronary Veins

The coronary (cardiac) veins travel alongside the arteries. Blood that has passed through the myocardial capillaries is drained by branches of the cardiac veins that join the coronary sinus.

The *coronary sinus* is the largest vein that drains the heart. It lies in the groove that separates the atria from the ventricles.

The Heart as a Pump

The heart functions as a pump to propel blood through the systemic and pulmonary circulations. As the heart chambers fill with blood, the heart muscle is stretched. The most important factor determining the amount of blood pumped by the heart is the amount of blood flowing into it from the systemic circulation (venous return).

Cardiac output is the amount of blood pumped into the aorta each minute by the heart. It is defined as the *stroke volume* (amount of blood ejected from a ventricle with each heartbeat) multiplied by the heart rate. In the average adult, normal cardiac output is between 4 and 8 L per minute. The cardiac output at rest is approximately 5 L per minute (stroke volume of 70 mL × a heart rate of 70 beats/min). Cardiac output may be increased by an increase in heart rate or stroke volume. Signs and symptoms of decreased cardiac output include cold, clammy skin; color changes in the skin and mucous membranes; dyspnea, orthopnea, and crackles (rales); changes in mental status; changes in blood pressure; dysrhythmias; jugular venous distention; fatigue; and restlessness.

Types of Cardiac Cells

In general, cardiac cells have either a mechanical *(contractile)* or an electrical *(pacemaker)* function (Table 1-2). Myocardial cells (working or mechanical cells) contain contractile filaments. When these cells are electrically stimulated, these filaments

TABLE **1-2**	**Types of Cardiac Cells**	
Type of Cardiac Cell	**Where Found**	**Primary Function**
Myocardial cells	Myocardium	Contraction and relaxation
Pacemaker cells	Conduction system	Generation and conduction of electrical impulses

slide together and the myocardial cell contracts. These myocardial cells form the muscular layer of the atrial walls and the thicker muscular layer of the ventricular walls *(the myocardium)*. Normally these cells do not spontaneously generate electrical impulses. Instead, they depend on pacemaker cells for this function. *Pacemaker cells* are specialized cells of the electrical conduction system responsible for the spontaneous generation and conduction of electrical impulses.

Cardiac Action Potential

> For electrical current to be generated, a difference between electrical charges must exist.

All living cells maintain a difference in the concentrations of ions across their cell membranes. Electrical impulses are the result of brief but rapid flow of charged particles (ions) back and forth across the cell membrane. The exchange of electrolytes in myocardial cells creates electrical activity, which appears on the ECG as waveforms. The major electrolytes that affect cardiac function are sodium (Na^+), potassium (K^+), and calcium (Ca^{2+}).

Depolarization and Repolarization

When the cardiac muscle cell is stimulated, the cell is said to *depolarize*. The inside of the cell becomes more positive because of the entry of Na^+ ions into the cell. Depolarization proceeds from the innermost layer of the heart *(endocardium)* to the outermost layer *(epicardium)*. On the ECG, the P wave represents atrial depolarization and the QRS complex represents ventricular depolarization.

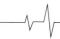

After the cell depolarizes, diffusion of Na⁺ into the cell stops. K⁺ is allowed to diffuse out of the cell, leaving negatively charged ions *(anions)* inside the cell. The cell returns to its resting level. This causes the contractile proteins to separate *(relax)*. The cell can then be stimulated again if another electrical impulse arrives at the cell membrane. Repolarization proceeds from the epicardium to the endocardium. On the ECG, the ST-segment and T wave represent ventricular repolarization.

Conduction System

The specialized electrical (pacemaker) cells in the heart are arranged in a system of pathways called the *conduction system* (Figure 1-4).

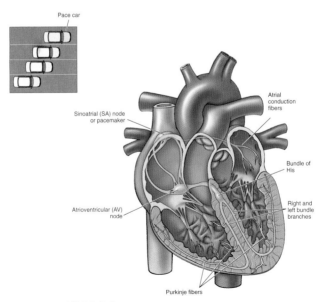

FIGURE **1-4** The heart's conduction system.

The normal heartbeat is the result of an electrical impulse that originates in the sinoatrial (sinus or SA) node. The SA node is located in the upper posterior portion of the right atrium at the junction of the superior vena cava and the right atrium. Because the cells of the SA node normally depolarize more rapidly than other cardiac cells, it is usually the primary pacemaker of the heart. The SA node initiates electrical impulses at a rhythmic rate of 60 to 100 beats/min.

As the impulse leaves the SA node, it is spread from cell to cell across the atrial muscle, depolarizing the right atrium, the interatrial septum, and then the left atrium, resulting in almost simultaneous contraction of the right and left atria. The impulse passes through the atrial muscle to the AV node by means of internodal pathways. Depolarization and repolarization are slow in the AV node, making this area vulnerable to blocks in conduction (AV blocks). The AV junction (the AV node and the nonbranching portion of the bundle of His) consists of specialized conduction tissue that provides the electrical links between the atrium and ventricle.

After passing through the AV node, the impulse enters the bundle of His. The *bundle of His* is located in the upper portion of the interventricular septum and connects the AV node with the right and left bundle branches. The bundle of His has pacemaker cells capable of discharging at a rate of 40 to 60 beats/min. The right bundle branch innervates the right ventricle. The left bundle branch spreads the electrical impulse to the interventricular septum and left ventricle, which is thicker and more muscular than the right ventricle. The left bundle branch divides into three divisions *(fascicles):* the *anterior fascicle, posterior fascicle,* and *septal fascicle.* The anterior fascicle spreads the electrical impulse to the anterior (superior) portions of the left ventricle. The posterior fascicle relays the impulse to the posterior (inferior) portions of the left ventricle, and the septal fascicle relays the impulse to the midseptum.

The right and left bundle branches divide into smaller and smaller branches and then into a special network of fibers called the *Purkinje fibers*. These fibers spread from the interventricular septum into the papillary muscles and then continue downward to the apex of the heart, making up an elaborate web that penetrates about one third of the way into the ventricular muscle mass. The fibers then become continuous with the muscle cells of the right and left ventricles. The Purkinje fibers have an intrinsic pacemaker ability of 20 to 40 beats/min.

CHAPTER 2

Introduction to the 12-Lead ECG

Electrocardiogram

The electrocardiogram (ECG) records the electrical activity of a large mass of atrial and ventricular cells as specific waveforms and complexes. The electrical activity within the heart can be observed by means of electrodes connected by cables to an ECG machine. Think of the ECG as a voltmeter that records the electrical voltages *(potentials)* generated by depolarization of heart muscle. The basic function of the ECG is to detect current flow as measured on the patient's skin. The ECG does *not* provide information about the mechanical *(contractile)* condition of the myocardium. The effectiveness of the heart's mechanical activity is evaluated by assessment of the patient's pulse and blood pressure.

Electrodes

Electrodes are applied at specific locations on the patient's chest and extremities to view the heart's electrical activity from different angles and planes. One end of a monitoring cable is attached to the electrode and the other end to an ECG machine.

Lead Placement

A lead is a record *(tracing)* of electrical activity between two electrodes. Each lead records the average current flow at a specific time in a portion of the heart. Leads allow viewing the heart's electrical activity in two different planes: frontal (coronal) and horizontal (transverse). Frontal plane leads view the heart from the front of the body. Horizontal plane leads view the heart as if the body were sliced in half horizontally. A 12-lead ECG provides views of the heart in both the frontal and horizontal planes and views the surfaces of the left ventricle from 12 different angles.

The standard 12-lead is composed of six limb leads and six chest leads (Table 2-1). Leads I, II, III, aVR, aVL, and aVF are obtained from electrodes placed on the patient's arms and legs. As their names suggest, the six chest leads, V_1 through V_6, are obtained from electrodes placed on the patient's chest. All 12 leads are obtained from only 10 electrodes (Figure 2-1). This is possible because the four limb electrodes are used for different purposes in different leads. For example, the left arm electrode is used as a negative electrode when lead III is obtained and is used as a positive electrode when lead aVL is obtained.

TABLE **2-1**	**Comparison of Various Leads**	
I, II, III	Limb lead	Bipolar
aVR, aVL, aVF	Limb lead	Unipolar
V_1, V_2, V_3, V_4, V_5, V_6	Chest lead	Unipolar

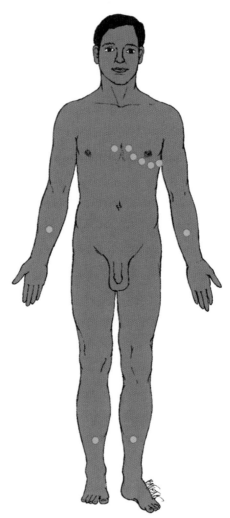

FIGURE **2-1** In a standard 12-lead ECG, all 12 leads are obtained from ten electrodes positioned as shown here.

Limb Leads

Leads I, II, and III make up the standard limb leads. Proper position requires that the electrodes for these leads be placed on the patient's limbs. The deltoid area is suitable for electrodes attached to the arms and is easily accessed. Either the thigh or the lower leg is suitable for the leg electrodes. Because each of these three leads has a distinct negative pole and a distinct positive pole, they are considered *bipolar.* The positive electrode is located at the left wrist in lead I; leads II and III both have their positive electrode located at the left foot. Each lead measures the difference in electrical potential between the positive pole and its corresponding negative.

Leads aVR, aVL, and aVF are augmented limb leads. The ECG machine augments (magnifies) the amplitude of the electrical potentials detected at each extremity by approximately 50% over those recorded at the bipolar leads. The "a" in aVR, aVL, and aVF refers to augmented. The "V" refers to voltage. The position of the positive electrode corresponds to the last letter in each of these leads. The positive pole in aVR is located on the right arm, aVL has a positive pole at the left arm, and aVF has a positive electrode positioned on the left leg.

Although leads aVR, aVL, and aVF have a distinct positive pole, they do not have a distinct negative pole. Because they have only one true pole, they are referred to as *unipolar leads*. In place of a single negative pole, these leads have multiple negative poles, creating a negative field *(central terminal)*, of which the heart is at the center (Figure 2-2). Theoretically, this makes the heart the negative electrode.

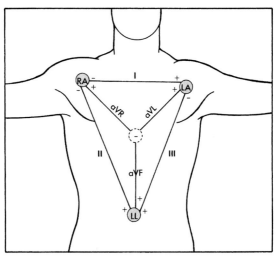

FIGURE **2-2** View of the standard limb leads and augmented limb leads.

Chest Leads

The six chest leads are identified as V_1, V_2, V_3, V_4, V_5, and V_6. Because the chest leads (also known as precordial leads) are unipolar, the positive electrode for each lead is placed at a specific location on the chest, and the heart is the theoretical negative electrode. The location of each lead is displayed in Figure 2-3.

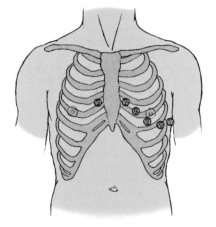

FIGURE **2-3** The position of the six chest (precordial) leads.

Other chest leads that are not part of a standard 12-lead ECG may be used to view specific surfaces of the heart. When a right ventricular myocardial infarction is suspected, right chest leads are used. Placement of right chest leads is identical to placement of the standard chest leads except it is done on the right side of the chest (Figure 2-4).

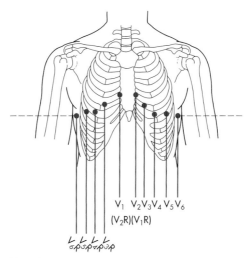

V_1 $V_2V_3V_4$ $V_5 V_6$
$(V_2R)(V_1R)$

FIGURE **2-4** Placement of the left and right chest leads.

What Each Lead "Sees"

Each positive electrode can be thought of as a camera or an eye looking in at the heart. Because the ECG does not directly measure the heart's electrical activity, it does not "see" all the current flowing through it. What the ECG does see from its vantage point on the body's surface is the net result of countless individual currents competing in a tug-of-war. For example, the QRS complex, which represents ventricular depolarization, is not a display of all the electrical activity occurring in the right and left ventricles. It is the net result of a tug-of-war produced by the numerous individual currents in both the right and left ventricles. Because the left ventricle is much more massive than the right, the left overpowers the right. What is seen in the QRS complex is the remaining electrical activity of the left ventricle, that is, the portion not used to cancel out the right ventricle. Therefore, in a normally conducted beat, the QRS complex represents the electrical activity occurring in the left ventricle.

The position of the positive electrode on the body determines which portion of the left ventricle is seen by each lead. The view of each lead is listed in Table 2-2; Figure 2-5 demonstrates the portion of the left ventricle that each lead views.

TABLE 2-2	What Each Lead "Sees"
Leads	**Heart Surface Viewed**
II, III, aVF	Inferior
V_1, V_2	Septal
V_3, V_4	Anterior
I, aVL, V_5, V_6	Lateral

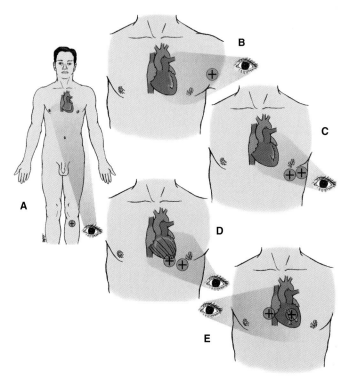

FIGURE **2-5** **A,** Leads II, III, and aVF each have their positive electrode positioned on the left leg. From the perspective of the left leg, each of them "sees" the inferior wall of the left ventricle. **B,** From their vantage point on the left arm, leads I and aVL "look" in at the lateral wall of the left ventricle. **C,** Leads V_5 and V_6 also "view" the lateral wall because they are positioned on the axillary area of the left chest. **D,** Leads V_3 and V_4 are positioned in the area of the anterior chest. From this perspective, these leads "see" the anterior wall of the left ventricle. **E,** The septal wall is "seen" by leads V_1 and V_2, which are positioned next to the sternum.

If an electrical impulse (wave of depolarization) moves toward the positive electrode, the waveform recorded on ECG graph paper will be upright (positive deflection). If the wave of depolarization moves toward the negative electrode, the waveform recorded will be inverted (downward or negative deflection). A biphasic (partly positive, partly negative) waveform or a straight line is recorded when the wave of depolarization moves perpendicularly to the positive electrode (Figure 2-6). Each waveform produced is related to a specific electrical event in the heart. When electrical activity is not detected, a straight line is recorded, called the *baseline* or *isoelectric line.*

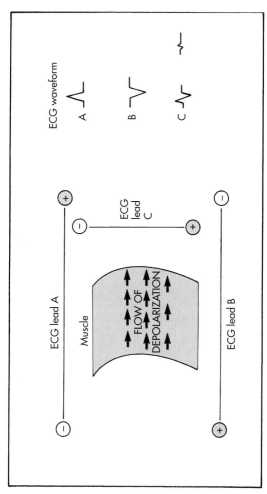

FIGURE 2-6 A, If an electrical impulse (wave of depolarization) moves toward the *positive* electrode, the waveform recorded on the ECG graph paper will be upright. B, If the wave of depolarization moves toward the *negative* electrode, the waveform produced will be inverted. C, A biphasic (partly positive, partly negative) waveform is recorded when the wave of depolarization moves perpendicularly to the positive electrode.

ECG Paper

Time

Electrocardiographic paper is graph paper made up of small and large boxes measured in millimeters (Figure 2-7). The smallest boxes are 1 mm wide and 1 mm high. The horizontal axis of the paper corresponds with time. ECG paper normally records at a constant speed of 25 mm per second. Thus each horizontal unit (1-mm box) represents 0.04 seconds (25 mm/sec × 0.04 sec = 1 mm). The lines between every five small boxes on the paper are heavier and indicate one large box. Because each large box is the width of five small boxes, a large box represents 0.20 seconds.

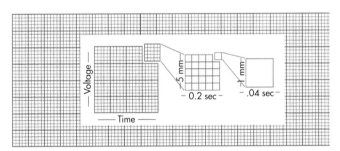

FIGURE **2-7** This example of ECG graph paper shows the relationship between time and voltage and the units used to measure them.

The 12-lead ECG provides only a 2.5-second view of each lead. When looking for evidence of infarction, most of the information is obtained from analyzing a single representative complex in each lead. It is assumed that 2.5 seconds is long enough to capture at least one representative complex. However, a 2.5-second view is not long enough to assess rate and rhythm properly, so at least one continuous rhythm strip is usually included at the bottom of the tracing.

Voltage

The *vertical axis* of the graph paper represents voltage or amplitude of the ECG waveforms or deflections. Voltage may appear as a positive or negative value because voltage is a force with direction as well as amplitude. The size or amplitude of a waveform is measured in millivolts (mV) or millimeters (mm).

Format of the 12-lead ECG

The most common format for displaying the 12-lead ECG is shown in Figure 2-8.

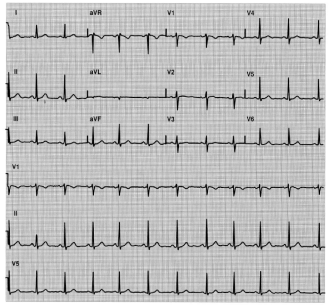

FIGURE **2-8** A sample 12-lead ECG.

Waveforms, Segments, Complexes, and Intervals

Electrical impulses originating in the SA node produce various waves on the ECG as they spread throughout the heart. The first wave in the cardiac cycle is the P wave. It represents atrial depolarization and the spread of the electrical impulse throughout the right and left atria. The *PR-segment* is part of the PR interval and is the horizontal line between the end of the P wave and the beginning of the QRS complex. The PR-segment is normally isoelectric. The P wave plus the PR-segment equals the *PR interval* (PRI). The PRI reflects depolarization of the right and left atria and the spread of the impulse through the AV node, bundle of His, right and left bundle branches, and Purkinje fibers. In adults, the PR interval normally measures 120 to 200 ms (0.12 to 0.20 sec).

The QRS complex consists of the Q wave, R wave, and S wave and represents the spread of the electrical impulse through the ventricles (ventricular depolarization). Depolarization triggers contraction of ventricular tissue. Thus, shortly after the QRS complex begins, the ventricles contract. A QRS complex normally follows each P wave. One or even two of the three waveforms that make up the QRS complex may not always be present.

The QRS complex begins as a downward deflection, the Q wave. A Q wave, if present, is **always** a negative waveform. The Q wave represents depolarization of the interventricular septum, which is activated from left to right. It is important to differentiate physiologic Q waves (present as a normal part of the QRS) from pathologic Q waves (Figure 2-9). A normal Q wave in the limb leads is less than 40 ms (less than 0.04 seconds, or one small box) in duration and less than one third the amplitude of the R wave in that lead. An abnormal (pathologic) Q wave is more than 40 ms (0.04 seconds) in duration and equal to or more than one third of the amplitude of the following R wave in that lead. Because myocardial infarction is a possible cause of Q waves, the duration and amplitude of every Q wave noted on the ECG should be examined.

The R wave is the first positive (upright) waveform following the P wave. The S wave is the negative waveform following the R wave. The R and S waves represent simultaneous

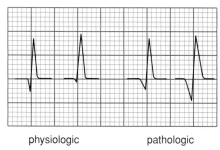

physiologic   pathologic

FIGURE **2-9** Physiologic and pathologic Q waves.

depolarization of the right and left ventricles. The QRS duration is a measurement of the time required for ventricular activation. QRS duration is most accurately determined when it is viewed and measured in more than one lead. The measurement should be taken from the QRS complex with the longest duration and clearest onset and end. The beginning of the QRS complex is measured from the point where the first wave of the complex begins to deviate from the baseline. The point at which the last wave of the complex begins to level out or distinctly change direction at, above, or below the baseline marks the end of the QRS complex. In adults, the normal duration of the QRS complex varies between 60 and 100 ms (0.06 and 0.10 seconds). If an electrical impulse does not follow the normal ventricular conduction pathway, it will take longer to depolarize the myocardium. Of course, this delay in conduction through the ventricle produces a wider QRS complex.

The portion of the ECG tracing between the QRS complex and the T wave is the ST-segment. The point where the QRS complex and the ST-segment meet is called the *junction*, or *J-point* (Figure 2-10). It may be difficult to determine the J-point clearly. The ST-segment represents the early part of repolarization of the right and left ventricles. The normal ST-segment begins at the isoelectric line, extends from the end of the S wave, and curves gradually upward to the beginning of the T wave. ST-segment depression is deviation of the segment below the baseline. ST-segment elevation is deviation of the segment above the baseline. Although some deviation of the ST-segment from the isoelectric line can be a normal finding, ST-segment

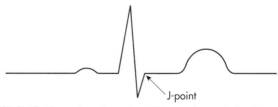

J-point

FIGURE **2-10** The point where the QRS complex and the ST-segment meet is called the *junction* or *J-point.*

elevation or depression is considered "significant" if the displacement is more than 1 mm (one box) and is seen in two or more leads facing the same anatomic area of the heart (also known as *contiguous leads*). Even if ST-segment changes are less than 1 mm, clinical data should be considered for the diagnosis of infarction. Myocardial ischemia, injury, and infarction are among the causes of ST-deviation.

Ventricular repolarization is represented on the ECG by the T wave. The beginning of the T wave is identified as the point where the slope of the ST-segment appears to become abruptly or gradually steeper. The T wave ends when it returns to the baseline. It may be difficult to determine the onset and end of the T wave clearly.

The QT interval encompasses the QRS complex, ST-segment, and T wave and represents total ventricular activity: the time from ventricular depolarization *(activation)* to repolarization *(recovery)*. The QT interval is measured from the beginning of the QRS complex to the end of the T wave. The duration of the QT interval varies according to age, gender, and particularly heart rate. A prolonged QT interval indicates a lengthened relative refractory period, which puts the ventricles at risk for life-threatening dysrhythmias, such as Torsade de Pointes.

A U wave is a small waveform that, when it is seen, follows the T wave. The mechanism of the U wave is not definitely known. One theory suggests that it represents repolarization of the Purkinje fibers. U waves are most easily seen when the heart rate is slow. Figure 2-11 displays the ECG waveforms, and Figure 2-12 displays the principal ECG intervals discussed in this chapter.

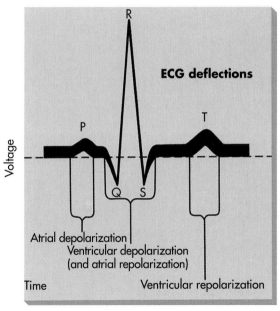

FIGURE **2-11** ECG waveforms: P, QRS, and T.

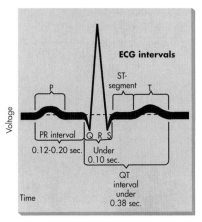

FIGURE **2-12** ECG segments and intervals: PR interval, QRS duration, ST-segment, QT interval.

Axis Deviation

Leads have a negative (-) and positive (+) electrode pole that senses the magnitude and direction of the electrical force caused by the spread of waves of depolarization and repolarization throughout the myocardium. A vector (arrow) is a symbol representing this force. Leads that face the tip or point of a vector record a positive deflection on ECG paper.

A mean vector identifies the average of depolarization waves in one portion of the heart. The mean P vector represents the average magnitude and direction of both right and left atrial depolarization. The mean QRS vector represents the average magnitude and direction of both right and left ventricular depolarization. The average direction of a mean vector is called the *mean axis* and is identified only in the frontal plane. Electrical axis refers to determining the direction (or angle in degrees) in which the main vector of depolarization is pointed.

During normal ventricular depolarization, the left side of the interventricular septum is stimulated first. The electrical impulse then crosses the septum to stimulate the right side. The left and right ventricles are then depolarized simultaneously. Because the left ventricle is considerably larger than the right, right ventricular depolarization forces are overshadowed on the ECG. As a result, the mean QRS vector points down (inferior) and to the left.

The axes of leads I, II, and III form an equilateral triangle with the heart at the center. If the augmented limb leads are added to this configuration and the axes of the six leads moved in a way in which they bisect each other, the result is the hexaxial reference system (Figure 2-13).

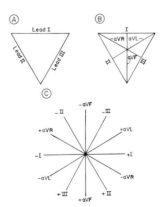

FIGURE **2-13** **A,** Einthoven's equilateral triangle formed by leads I, II, and III. **B,** The unipolar leads are added to the equilateral triangle. **C,** The hexaxial reference system derived from B.

The hexaxial reference system represents all of the frontal plane (limb) leads with the heart in the center and is the means used to express the location of the frontal plane axis. This system forms a 360-degree circle surrounding the heart. The positive end of lead I is designated at 0 degrees. The six frontal plane leads divide the circle into segments, each representing 30 degrees. All degrees in the upper hemisphere are labeled as *negative degrees,* and all degrees in the lower hemisphere are labeled as *positive degrees.* The mean QRS vector (normal electrical axis) lies between 0 and +90 degrees.

Current flow to the right of normal is called *right axis deviation* (+90 to +180 degrees). Current flow in the direction opposite of normal is called *indeterminate, "no man's land," northwest,* or *extreme right axis deviation* (−91 to −179 degrees). Current flow to the left of normal is called *left axis deviation* (−1 to −90 degrees).

In the hexaxial reference system, the axes of some leads are perpendicular to each other. Lead I is perpendicular to lead aVF. Lead II is perpendicular to aVL, and lead III is perpendicular to lead aVR. If the electrical force moves toward a positive electrode, a positive (upright) deflection will be recorded. If the electrical force moves away from a positive electrode, a negative (downward) deflection will be recorded. If the electrical force is parallel to a given lead, the largest deflection in that lead will be recorded. If the electrical force is perpendicular to a lead axis, the resulting ECG complex will be small or biphasic in that lead.

Leads I and aVF divide the heart into four quadrants. These two leads can be used to estimate electrical axis quickly. In leads I and aVF, the QRS complex is normally positive. If the QRS complex in either or both of these leads is negative, axis deviation is present (Table 2-3).

TABLE **2-3**	Two-Lead Method of Axis Determination			
Axis	**Normal**	**Left**	**Right**	**Indeterminate ("no man's land")**
Lead I—QRS direction	Positive	Positive	Negative	Negative
Lead aVF—QRS direction	Positive	Negative	Positive	Negative

CHAPTER 3

Acquiring the 12-Lead ECG

Goals

Acquisition of a 12-lead ECG should be clear, accurate, and fast:

* *Clear.* The baseline is steady, and the tracing is free of artifact.
* *Accurate.* The leads are applied correctly, and the monitor is properly configured to obtain a diagnostic-quality ECG.
* *Fast.* The entire process should not be time consuming or delay patient treatment.

Clear

Accurate 12-lead ECG interpretation requires a tracing in which the waveforms and intervals are free of distortion. Distortion of an ECG tracing by electrical activity that is noncardiac in origin is called *artifact*. One of the methods you can use to reduce artifact is to help the electrode gel penetrate the patient's skin. If the gel can penetrate the skin well, the result is an increased signal strength and reduced artifact.

Proper preparation of the patient's skin and evaluation of the equipment (electrodes, wires) before use can minimize the problems associated with artifact.

Accurate

Lead Placement

Each lead of a standard 12-lead ECG correlates with a specific anatomic region of the left ventricle. An accurate 12-lead requires placing the electrodes correctly, positioning the patient, and selecting the correct settings for a diagnostic quality tracing.

The following are the standard locations for limb lead electrodes:

- Right arm electrode on the inside of the patient's right wrist
- Left arm electrode on the inside of the patient's left wrist
- Left leg electrode on the inner aspect of the patient's left leg near the ankle
- Right leg electrode on the inner aspect of the patient's right ankle

Proper placement of the chest leads requires the ability to pinpoint specific anatomic locations, particularly certain intercostal spaces. Various landmarks can be used to determine the correct location of these intercostal spaces. The particular method used is of little consequence as long as the leads are properly located. The key is to correctly position V_1, which lies in the fourth intercostal space. A summary of the chest leads is shown in Table 3-1.

TABLE 3-1	Summary of Chest Leads	
Lead	**Positive Electrode Position**	**Heart Surface Viewed**
V_1	Right side of sternum, 4th intercostal space	Septum
V_2	Left side of sternum, 4th intercostal space	Septum
V_3	Midway between V_2 and V_4	Anterior
V_4	Left midclavicular line, 5th intercostal space	Anterior
V_5	Left anterior axillary line at same level as V_4	Lateral
V_6	Left midaxillary line at same level as V_4	Lateral

The right ventricle and the posterior wall of the left ventricle are not "seen" by the standard 12-lead ECG. To identify infarction in these areas, extra leads are required. When obtaining right-sided or posterior leads, a standard 12-lead is obtained first. The cables for the standard V leads are then moved to the electrodes for the additional leads. Any V-lead cable can be moved to obtain the right or posterior leads. Once these leads are printed, however, the correct lead must be handwritten onto the ECG to indicate the origin of the tracing (Figure 3-1). The computer-generated interpretation must also be disregarded in the event that the cables have been moved.

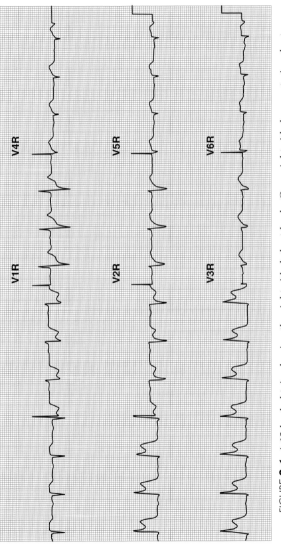

FIGURE **3-1** A 12-lead obtained using the right-sided or posterior chest leads are printed, the correct lead must be handwritten onto the ECG.

Placement of right chest leads is identical to placement of the standard chest leads except it is done on the right side of the chest (Figure 3-2). The following are the right chest leads and their placement:

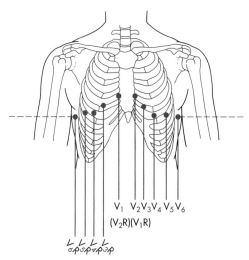

FIGURE **3-2** Placement of the left and right chest leads.

- Lead V_1R = Lead V_2
- Lead V_2R = Lead V_1
- Lead V_3R = Midway between V_2R and V_4R
- Lead V_4R = Right midclavicular line, fifth intercostal space
- Lead V_5R = Right anterior axillary line at same level as V_4R
- Lead V_6R = Right midaxillary line at same level as V_4R

The leads corresponding to the posterior wall of the left ventricle are V_7, V_8, and V_9. These three leads are positioned horizontally level with V_4. Lead V_7 is placed at the posterior axillary line. Lead V_8 is placed at the angle of the scapula (posterior scapular line), and lead V_9 is placed over the left border of the spine. The position for these leads is shown in Figure 3-3.

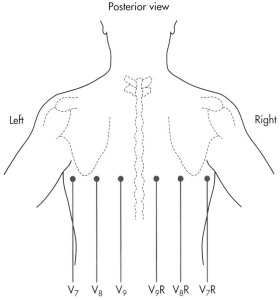

Posterior view

Left

Right

V_7 V_8 V_9 V_9R V_8R V_7R

FIGURE **3-3** Posterior chest lead placement.

Frequency Response

The spectrum in which an ECG can accurately reproduce the signals it is sensing is referred to as the *frequency response.* Monitors may be designed with either a narrow or wide frequency response. Each has its advantages and disadvantages.

Frequency response can be considered the window through which the ECG looks. If the window is large, the ECG sees a lot; if the window is smaller, the ECG sees less. Which is better? The answer depends on the purpose for which the ECG monitor is being used. If rate and rhythm are the primary objective, a narrow frequency response is desirable. The narrow frequency response does not let the monitor see much of the artifact and noise that can produce an unclear tracing. This simplifies the process of locating P waves, measuring intervals, and all the other aspects of rhythm assessment. However, as helpful as a narrow frequency response can be when determining rate and rhythm, recognition of the ECG changes associated with acute coronary syndromes requires a wide frequency response. A narrow frequency response can be referred to as *monitor quality* and a wide frequency response can be referred to as *diagnostic quality*. Figure 3-4 demonstrates how changes in frequency response affect what the monitor can and cannot see.

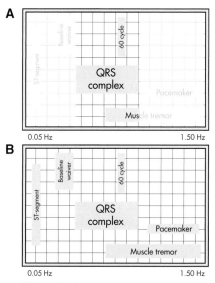

FIGURE **3-4 A,** With a limited frequency response the monitor can clearly "see" the QRS complex but cannot see the other features as clearly. **B,** With a wider frequency response, the monitor can "see" the QRS complex and the ST-segment as well.

Calibration

The significance of standard calibration is moot when the monitor is used only to determine rate and rhythm. However, proper calibration is critical when analyzing ST-segments.

The cardiac monitor's sensitivity to electrical current is variable. When the sensitivity is increased, a larger complex is produced. Likewise, a smaller complex is the result of decreased sensitivity. The button or control that adjusts the monitor's sensitivity can be labelled with a variety of names, some of which are ECG size, sensitivity, gain, and calibration. The standard for ECG recording is 1 mV = 10 mm. This means that when an ECG monitor is in standard calibration, a 10-mm (two big boxes) deflection is produced for every millivolt that is sensed (Figure 3-5).

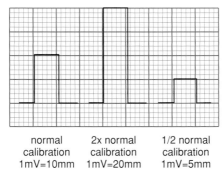

normal	2x normal	1/2 normal
calibration	calibration	calibration
1mV=10mm	1mV=20mm	1mV=5mm

FIGURE **3-5** The size of the ECG may be adjusted as needed. However, ST-segment analysis must be adjusted accordingly whenever non-standard calibration is used.

Paper Speed

The rate at which the paper goes through the printer is adjustable and is designated on the 12-lead. Standard paper speed is 25 mm per second. A faster paper speed makes the rhythm appear slower and the QRS wider. Thus in cases of tachycardia a faster paper speed makes it easier to see the waveforms and analyze the tachycardia. A slower paper speed makes the rhythm appear faster and the QRS narrower.

Fast

When treating cardiac patients, much has to be accomplished in a short time. Fortunately, a 12-lead can be obtained very quickly, even in these circumstances. Just as with virtually every other skill, 12-lead acquisition can be done more quickly with practice. Practice should be gained with various body types and both genders. In addition to practice, another tip is to apply the limb electrodes whenever you think a 12-lead might be done. Clearly not every patient that you monitor will need a 12-lead. However, if you have already placed the limb leads on the limbs and not the torso, they can be used for both rhythm monitoring and a diagnostic 12-lead ECG. Another tip is to remove the patient's clothes from the waist up. Of course, the patient's modesty must be maintained with a gown, sheet, or towel.

12-Lead Acquisition

Once the electrodes have been properly positioned, the cables can be attached. With a 12-lead monitor, it is simply a matter of following the manufacturer's instructions and pushing the right button(s) to record the tracing. Most 12-lead monitors record all 12 leads simultaneously but display them in the conventional three row by four column format. Therefore, all the QRS complexes in a row are consecutive, whereas QRS complexes that are aligned vertically represent a simultaneous recording of the same beat (Figure 3-6). Because the leads are obtained simultaneously, only 10 seconds of sampling time is required to record all 12 leads.

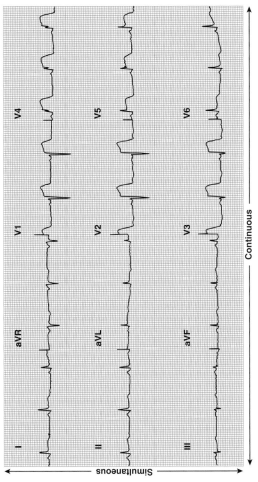

FIGURE **3-6** In a simultaneous tracing, the beats in a vertical column are all the product of the same ventricular contraction. Likewise, beats in a horizontal row are continuous, even as the leads change.

Troubleshooting

The presence of artifact can interfere with a 12-lead machine's ability to acquire or interpret the ECG. Consider the following possible causes of artifact or baseline wander.

Equipment-related Causes

ECG Electrodes
Always use fresh electrodes when obtaining a 12-lead ECG. If the electrode gel has dried out, it is not able to penetrate the skin. If the gel does not penetrate the skin, the signal to the monitor is weak and artifact results.

Loose, Cracked, or Damaged Cables
The signal from the patient's heart is conducted through the cables to the monitor. If the cable's insulation is cracked or if a lead wire is damaged, the signal to the monitor is affected and artifact can result. Check and reconnect the cable connections. Inspect the cables and replace them if they are damaged.

Technique-related Causes

Patient Movement
When the position of the baseline is in a state of flux, ST-segment analysis is very difficult. As the baseline wanders, the isoelectric point changes from moment to moment. In this situation, the J-point, though it may have been isoelectric when inscribed, can appear elevated above the PR and TP segments, as shown in Figure 3-7. This ST-segment elevation may not be the result of infarction, but it rather may be simply an expected finding that occurs as the monitor centers the isoelectric line in the screen. Therefore, be very cautious about analyzing ST-segment elevation in leads with a wandering baseline. If an ECG is being obtained via a standard monitor, wait until the tracing is centered for several beats before moving to the next lead.

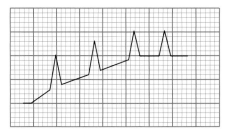

FIGURE **3-7** The J-point is isoelectric, but compared with the TP and PR-segments, it appears elevated. Note that when the baseline returns to the centered position, the ST-segment no longer appears elevated. Do not perform ST-segment analysis in this situation.

A common cause of a wandering baseline is patient movement. Subtle patient movements, such as that caused by the patient's respirations, talking, shivering, tapping their toes, or rolling their fingers, can be enough to produce artifact. When the tracing quality precludes a good interpretation, the tracing should be repeated. Efforts made to reduce muscle tension and the source of patient movement, such as having the patient relax and take a deep breath before acquisition, can improve the tracing quality.

Cable Movement
Cable movement is another possible cause of artifact. The cables may tug on the electrodes or pull away from the patient. Many manufacturers provide a cable clasp to secure the cable assembly during acquisition. Secure the cable by clipping the cable clasp to the sheet or the patient's clothing.

Vehicle Movement
Many Emergency Medical Services (EMS) professionals are able to obtain a clear ECG in a moving vehicle. However, it may be necessary to wait for the vehicle to stop at a traffic light or even pull over to acquire a clear ECG. Once the electrodes have been

placed and the cable is attached, 12-lead acquisition takes only 10 seconds.

Electromagnetic Interference

Some electrical devices may interfere with the 12-lead monitor. If artifact persists after removing hair and prepping the skin and normal troubleshooting did not turn up any problems, then think about electromagnetic interference (EMI). To correct the problem, ensure that power cords are not touching or lying near the ECG cable. Check for equipment that could be causing EMI (such as a radio transmitter or bed control). If such equipment is present, relocate or unplug the equipment that is causing the interference. Alternately, move the patient to a different area.

CHAPTER 4

Acute Coronary Syndromes

Acute coronary syndromes (ACSs) are a physiologic continuum of conditions caused by a similar sequence of pathologic events, that is, a transient or permanent obstruction of a coronary artery. ACSs include unstable angina, non-ST-segment elevation myocardial infarction (MI), and ST-segment elevation MI. These conditions are characterized by an excessive demand or inadequate supply of oxygen and nutrients to the heart muscle associated with plaque disruption, thrombus formation, and vasoconstriction. Sudden cardiac death can occur with any of these conditions.

Goals in the Immediate Management of Acute Coronary Syndromes

- Minimize infarct size.
- Salvage ischemic myocardium.
- Alleviate vasoconstriction.
- Reduce myocardial oxygen demand.
- Prevent and manage complications.
- Improve chances of survival.

49

Coronary Artery Obstruction

The usual cause of an ACS is the rupture of an atherosclerotic plaque. *Arteriosclerosis* is a chronic disease of the arterial system characterized by abnormal thickening and hardening of the vessel walls. *Atherosclerosis* is a form of arteriosclerosis in which the thickening and hardening of the vessel walls are caused by an accumulation of fatty deposits in the innermost lining of large and middle-sized muscular arteries. As fatty deposits build up, the opening of the artery gradually narrows and blood flow to the muscle decreases. A decreased supply of oxygenated blood to a body part or organ is called *ischemia.*

Atherosclerotic plaques differ in composition, consistency, vulnerability to rupture, and their tendency to generate a thrombus. Determinants of a plaque's vulnerability to rupture are thought to include the size of the lipid core and the thickness of the fibrous cap. "Stable" (i.e., unlikely to rupture) plaques are hard, consist primarily of collagen-rich sclerotic tissue, and have a thick fibrous cap over the lipid core that separates it from contact with the blood, making these plaques less likely to rupture (Figure 4-1). As these plaques increase in size, they can produce severe narrowing of the arterial lumen. A 70%-diameter stenosis is generally required to produce anginal symptoms. Complete occlusion of the vessel may cause infarction; however, because the plaque typically increases in size over months and years, collateral arteries may develop to supply tissue, thus preventing infarction despite complete vessel occlusion.

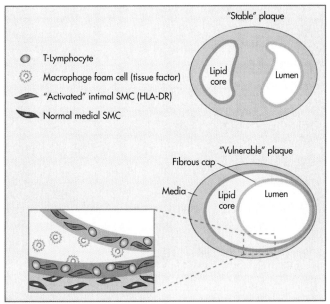

FIGURE **4-1** Comparison of "stable" and "vulnerable" plaques. A stable plaque has a relatively thick fibrous cap separating the lipid core from contact with the blood. A vulnerable plaque typically has a large lipid core and a thin cap of fibrous tissue that separates it from the vessel lumen. *SMC*, smooth muscle cell.

"Vulnerable" (prone to rupture) plaques are soft and have a thin cap of fibrous tissue over the lipid core that separates it from the vessel lumen (Figure 4-2). Vulnerable plaques tend to rupture at these cap regions where the atherosclerotic area of the artery lies next to the relatively normal part of the vessel wall. If the fibrous cap ruptures, the contents of the plaque (including collagen and other tissue factors) are exposed to flowing blood, which promotes platelet adhesion and

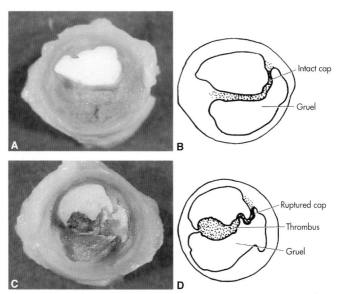

FIGURE **4-2** Macroscopic view of a vulnerable plaque. **A + B,** The yellow, soft atheromatous material ("gruel") is separated from the opening of the vessel only by a thin, but intact, fibrous cap. The vessel opening contains white radiographic contrast medium. **C + D,** This specimen was just a few millimeters distal to the one shown in A. Here the thin fibrous cap is ruptured, a big cap fragment and some of the soft atheromatous gruel are missing (due to downstream embolization), and a mural thrombus has evolved where the thrombogenic atheromatous gruel has been exposed. White contrast medium has penetrated the soft gruel through the ruptured cap.

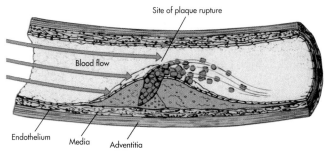

Site of plaque rupture

Blood flow

Endothelium   Media   Adventitia

FIGURE **4-3** Rupture of a vulnerable plaque results in adhesion of platelets at the site and activation of additional platelets (aggregation). The coagulation cascade then begins, resulting in additional platelet aggregation and thrombosis.

aggregation. The coagulation cascade then begins, resulting in additional platelet aggregation and thrombosis (Figure 4-3).

Occlusion of a coronary artery by a thrombus may be complete or incomplete. Complete occlusion of the coronary artery may result in ST-elevation MI (STEMI) or sudden death. Incomplete occlusion of the coronary artery by a thrombus may result in no clinical signs and symptoms (*silent MI*), unstable angina, non-ST-segment elevation MI (NSTEMI) or, possibly, sudden death.

The extent of arterial narrowing and the reduction in blood flow are critical determinants of coronary artery disease (CAD). The patient's clinical presentation and outcome depend on factors that include the following:

- Amount of myocardium supplied by the affected artery
- Severity and duration of myocardial ischemia
- Electrical instability of the ischemic myocardium
- Degree and duration of coronary obstruction
- Presence (and extent) or absence of collateral coronary circulation

Ischemia, Injury, and Infarction

Remember that the walls of the ventricles consist of an outer layer *(epicardium)*, middle layer *(myocardium)*, and an inner layer *(endocardium)* (Figure 4-4). The myocardium is subdivided into two areas. The innermost half of the myocardium is called the *subendocardial area;* the outermost half is called the *subepicardial area.* The main coronary arteries lie on the epicardial surface of

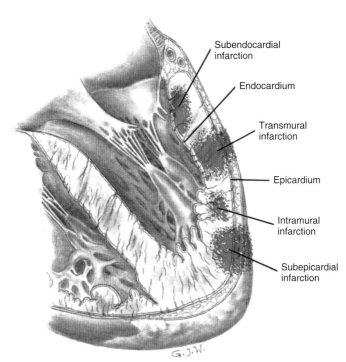

FIGURE **4-4** Possible locations of infarctions in the ventricular wall.

the heart (Figure 4-5) and feed this area first before supplying the heart's inner layers with oxygenated blood. The subendocardium is at greatest risk of ischemia because this area has a high demand for oxygen and is fed by the most distal branches of the coronary arteries.

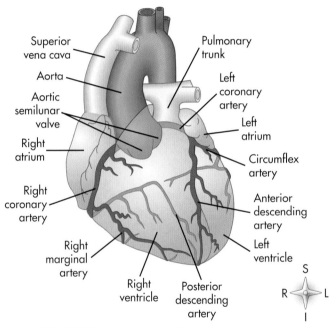

FIGURE **4-5** Anterior view of the coronary circulation.

Myocardial ischemia is the result of an imbalance between the metabolic needs of the myocardium (demand) and the flow of oxygenated blood to it (supply) (Table 4-1). Ischemia can occur because of increased myocardial oxygen demand (demand ischemia), reduced myocardial oxygen supply (supply ischemia), or both. Ischemia affects the heart's cells that are responsible for contraction as well as those responsible for generation and conduction of electrical impulses. These effects are related to delays in depolarization and repolarization and can be viewed on the ECG as transient changes in ST-segments and T waves. These ECG changes, and the chest pain or discomfort that accompanies myocardial ischemia, usually resolve when the demand for oxygen is reduced (by resting or slowing the heart rate with medications such as beta-blockers) to a level that can be supplied by the coronary artery or increasing blood flow by dilating the coronary arteries with medications such as nitroglycerin (NTG).

TABLE 4-1	Possible Causes of Myocardial Ischemia	
Inadequate Oxygen Supply	Increased Myocardial Oxygen Demand	
Anemia	Exercise	Cocaine, amphetamines
Hypoxemia	Smoking	Emotional stress
Coronary artery narrowing caused by a thrombus, vasospasm, or rapid progression of atherosclerosis	Eating a heavy meal	Hypertension
	Fever	Exposure to cold weather
	Congestive heart failure	Aortic stenosis
	Tachydysrhythmias	Pheochromocytoma
	Obstructive cardiomyopathy	Thyrotoxicosis

Ischemia prolonged more than just a few minutes results in myocardial injury. Injured myocardial cells are still alive but will *infarct* (die) if the ischemia is not quickly corrected. If blood flow is quickly restored, no tissue death occurs. Myocardial injury can be extensive enough to produce a decrease in pump function or electrical conductivity in the affected cells. Injured myocardial cells do not depolarize completely, remaining electrically more positive than the uninjured areas surrounding them. This is viewed on the ECG as ST-segment elevation in the leads facing the affected area.

An MI occurs when blood flow to the heart muscle stops or is suddenly decreased long enough to cause cell death. Infarcted cells are without function and cannot respond to an electrical stimulus or provide any mechanical function.

Angina

Angina pectoris is chest discomfort or other related symptoms caused by myocardial ischemia. If the process is not quickly reversed and blood flow restored, myocardial ischemia may lead to cellular injury and, ultimately, infarction. Angina is typically described as "pressing," "squeezing," "strangling," "constricting," "bursting," "burning," "a band across the chest," "a weight in the center of the chest," or a "vise tightening around the chest." Many patients describe angina as a discomfort or pressure, not a "pain." Common sites for anginal discomfort are shown in Figure 4-6.

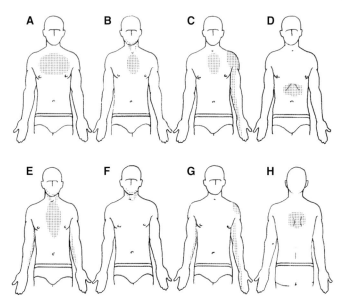

FIGURE **4-6** Common sites for anginal discomfort. **A,** Upper part
of chest. **B,** Beneath sternum radiating to the neck and jaw.
C, Beneath sternum radiating down left arm. **D,** Epigastric. **E,** Epigastric radiating to neck, jaw, and arms. **F,** Neck and jaw. **G,** Left shoulder.
H, Intrascapular.

Stable (Classic) Angina

Stable angina remains relatively constant and predictable in terms
of frequency of episodes, severity, duration, time of appearance,
precipitating factors, and response to therapy. It is characterized
by transient episodes of chest discomfort related to activities that
increase myocardial oxygen demand (e.g., emotional upset, exer-
cise/exertion, exposure to cold weather) and may be associated
with shortness of breath, palpitations, sweating, nausea, or vomiting. The duration of symptoms is typically 2 to 5 minutes and
occasionally 5 to 15 minutes. Prolonged discomfort (i.e., longer
than 30 minutes) is uncommon in stable angina.

Unstable Angina

Unstable angina is a syndrome of intermediate severity between stable angina and acute MI. Unlike stable angina, the discomfort associated with unstable angina may be described as painful. Unstable angina occurs most often in men and women 60 to 80 years of age who have one or more of the major risk factors for CAD (e.g., hypertension, hyperlipidemia, cigarette smoking, or diabetes mellitus) and is characterized by one or more of the following:

- Symptoms that occur at rest (or minimal exertion) and usually lasting longer than 20 minutes
- Symptoms that are severe or of new onset (i.e., within the previous 4 to 6 weeks)
- Symptoms that are more severe, prolonged, or frequent in a patient with preexisting stable angina

Unstable angina is associated with significant mortality. These patients should be treated as high-priority patients. During their initial presentation, distinguishing patients with unstable angina from those with acute MI is often impossible because their clinical presentations and ECG findings may be identical. Early assessment, including a focused history, and intervention are essential to prevent worsening ischemia. Serial ECGs and continuous ECG monitoring should be performed. Serum cardiac markers should be obtained on initial presentation to rule out infarction and again in 6 hours. If serum cardiac markers reveal evidence of myocardial necrosis, the diagnosis is NSTEMI.

Myocardial Infarction

In the strictest sense, the term *myocardial infarction* relates to necrosed myocardial tissue. In a practical sense, this term is applied to the *process* that results in the death of myocardial tissue. Consider the "process" of MI as a continuum rather than the presence of dead heart tissue. If efforts are made to recognize the process of MI, patients may be identified earlier and, if promptly treated, may altogether avoid the loss of myocardial tissue.

The diagnosis for an acute, evolving, or recent MI can be made with either of the following criteria:[1]

1. Typical rise and gradual fall (troponin) or more rapid rise and fall (CK-MB) of biochemical markers of myocardial necrosis with at least one of the following:
   a. Ischemic symptoms
   b. Development of pathologic Q waves on the ECG
   c. ECG changes indicative of ischemia (ST-segment elevation or depression)
   d. Coronary artery intervention (e.g., coronary angioplasty)
2. Pathologic findings of an acute MI

Once the process of tissue death begins, it continues quickly. The progress of tissue death has been described as a "wave" that begins in the endocardium and spreads to the epicardium. As the wave extends, the infarction becomes larger (Figure 4-7). The only way that the infarction can be halted is if the source of the coronary artery occlusion can be eliminated.

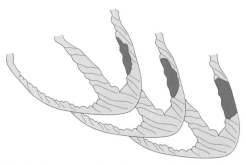

FIGURE **4-7** Wavefront expansion of myocardial infarction progresses from endocardium to epicardium.

Clinical Presentation

Chest discomfort suggestive of myocardial ischemia is the single most common symptom of infarction and is present in 75% to 80% of patients with acute MI. Symptoms frequently include chest, epigastric, arm, and wrist or jaw discomfort with exertion or at rest. The discomfort is typically described as heaviness, pressure, squeezing, or tightness in the chest that has persisted for at least 20 minutes, but it may be shorter in duration. Discomfort may begin in the central or left chest and then radiate to the arm, jaw, back, or shoulder. Symptoms may be accompanied by unexplained nausea and vomiting; persistent shortness of breath resulting from left ventricular failure; and unexplained weakness, dizziness, sweating, anxiety, lightheadedness, syncope, or a combination of these symptoms. Symptoms may occur with or without associated chest discomfort. Discomfort is usually not sharp, worsened by deep inspiration, affected by moving muscles in the area where the discomfort is localized, or positional in nature.

Atypical Presentation

Chest discomfort is absent in about 20% of patients experiencing an infarction. These patients are more likely to present with "anginal equivalent" symptoms or vague, nonspecific complaints. Patients more likely to present atypically include older adults, diabetic patients, and women.

Anginal equivalent symptoms are symptoms of myocardial ischemia other than chest pain or discomfort. Such symptoms include generalized weakness, dyspnea, excessive sweating, dizziness, syncope or near syncope, palpitations, fatigue, dysrhythmias, or exercise-induced pain in the abdominal region, back, jaw, arm, or shoulder.

The most frequent symptoms of acute MI in the older patients are shortness of breath, fatigue, and abdominal or epigastric discomfort. Older patients are more likely to have more severe preexisting conditions, such as hypertension, congestive heart failure, or previous acute MI; are likely to delay longer in seeking treatment compared with younger patients; and are less likely to have ST-segment elevation on their initial ECG.

Diabetic patients may present atypically (because of autonomic dysfunction) with generalized weakness, syncope, lightheadedness, or a change in mental status. Women who experience an ACS often describe their discomfort as aching, tightness, pressure, sharpness, burning, fullness, or tingling. The location of the discomfort is often in the back, shoulder, or neck. Some women have vague chest discomfort that tends to come and go with no known aggravating factors. Frequent acute symptoms include shortness of breath, weakness, unusual fatigue, cold sweats, dizziness, and nausea/vomiting.

ECG Changes

In the acute phase of an NSTEMI, the ST-segment may be depressed in the leads facing the surface of the infarcted area. NSTEMI can be diagnosed only if ST-segment and T-wave changes are accompanied by elevations of serum cardiac markers indicative of myocardial necrosis. Patients with NSTEMI are known to be at higher risk for death, reinfarction, and other morbidity than those with unstable angina. NSTEMIs tend to be smaller and have a better *short-term* prognosis than ST-elevation infarctions. However, the overall prognosis is similar to ST-elevation MIs. Recurrence of the infarct is common in the days to weeks after the patient has been sent home. This is referred to as *completion* of the infarction. Recent data suggest that the incidence of NSTEMI is increasing as the population of older patients with more advanced disease increases.

Most patients with ST-segment elevation will develop Q-wave MI. Only a minority of patients with ischemic chest discomfort at rest who do not have ST-segment elevation will develop a Q-wave MI. A Q-wave MI is diagnosed by the development of abnormal Q waves in serial ECGs. These infarctions tend to be larger than non-ST-segment elevation MIs, reflecting more damage to the left ventricle.

Recognition of infarction on the ECG relies on the detection of morphologic changes (i.e., changes in shape) of the QRS complex, the T wave, and the ST-segment. These changes occur in relation to certain events during the infarction. Figure 4-8 shows the ECG changes resulting from STEMI that often occur in a predictable pattern. The changes described below are not seen in every lead; they appear only in leads looking at the infarct site.

The first change you might detect in the ECG is the development of a tall T wave. In addition to an increase in height, the T wave becomes more symmetric and may become pointed (Figure 4-8, *A*). These T-wave changes may occur within the first few minutes of infarction, during what has been described as the *hyperacute phase* of infarction. As time progresses, signs of myocardial injury may develop. ST-segment elevation (Figure 4-8, *B*) provides the primary indication of myocardial injury in progress. ST-segment elevation may occur within the first hour or first few hours of infarction and is considered to occur in the early acute phase of infarction. In the later acute phase of the infarction, one may see the presence of T wave inversion, suggesting the presence of ischemia (Figure 4-8, *C*). In fact, T-wave inversion may precede the development of ST-segment elevation, or they may occur simultaneously.

A few hours later, the ECG may give its first evidence that tissue death has occurred. That evidence comes with the development of abnormal Q waves (Figure 4-8, *D*). Remember that a Q wave that is 40 ms or more wide (one small box or more wide) or more than one third the amplitude of the R wave in that lead is suggestive of infarction. An abnormal Q wave indicates the presence of dead myocardial tissue and, subsequently, a loss of electrical activity. Abnormal Q waves can appear within hours

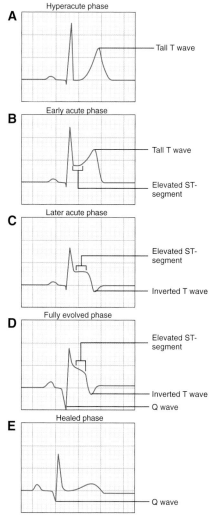

FIGURE **4-8** The evolving pattern of ST-elevation myocardial infarction on the ECG.

after occlusion of a coronary artery, but they more commonly appear several hours or days after the onset of signs and symptoms of an acute MI. When combined with ST-segment or T-wave changes, the presence of abnormal Q waves suggests an acute MI.

In time, the T wave regains its normal contour and the ST-segment returns to the isoelectric line. The Q wave, however, often remains as evidence that an infarct has occurred (Figure 4-8, *E*). When this pattern is seen, establishing the time of the infarct is impossible. It is only possible to recognize the presence of a previous MI.

The changes just described can be referred to as the indicative changes of MI. Of the indicative changes, ST-segment elevation is especially well suited for the detection of MI in the early hours. A tall T wave alone is not specific enough to diagnose MI, and T-wave inversion may occur in stable angina. Because a pathologic Q wave may take hours to develop to confirm the presence of MI (and not all MIs develop pathologic Q waves), the patient's signs and symptoms, serum cardiac markers, and the presence of ST-segment elevation provide the strongest evidence for the early recognition of MI.

Initial Assessment

If findings are consistent with a possible or definite ACS, the following interventions (including obtaining and reviewing a 12-lead ECG) should be performed within 10 minutes of patient presentation:

- Targeted history/physical examination; use a checklist (yes/no); focus on eligibility for reperfusion therapy.
  - Determine the patient's age, gender, signs and symptoms (including location of pain, duration, quality, relation to effort, and time of symptom onset), history of CAD, and presence of CAD risk factors.

- Assess vital signs, determine oxygen saturation.
- Establish intravenous (IV) access, ECG monitoring.
- Administer oxygen.
- Administer aspirin 162 to 325 mg (chewed) if no reason for exclusion.
- Obtain baseline serum cardiac marker levels.
- Obtain a 12-lead ECG.
  - Obtain first 12-lead ECG. Repeat with each set of vital signs, when the patient's symptoms change, and as often as necessary. Emergency departments should have an acute MI protocol that yields a targeted clinical examination and a 12-lead ECG within 10 minutes and a door-to-drug time that is less than 30 minutes.[2]
  - The provider reviewing the 12-lead should categorize the patient into one of four groups:
    1. T-wave inversion or normal ECG
    2. ST-segment elevation
    3. ST-segment depression
    4. Confounders (e.g., bundle branch block [BBB], left ventricular hypertrophy [LVH], or paced rhythm) where ischemia is difficult or impossible to interpret[3]
  - An absence of signs of ischemia on an ECG or in early laboratory data does not exclude the possibility of acute ischemia.
- Obtain serial ECGs in patients with a history suggesting MI and a nondiagnostic ECG.
- Obtain lab specimens (complete blood cell count [CBC], lipid profile, electrolytes).
- Portable chest x-ray, preferably upright.
- Administer NTG sublingual or spray.
  - Before administration, ensure IV access, systolic blood pressure > 90 mm Hg, heart rate > 50 beats/min, no right ventricular infarction, no use of Viagra, Cialis, or similar medication in previous 24 to 48 hours.
  - Administer morphine 2 to 4 mg IV for pain as needed.

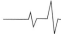

Interventions

Figure 4-9 was obtained from a chest pain patient before hospitalization. The prehospital 12-lead suggested the presence of acute MI, and the results of the reperfusion therapy checklist suggested that the patient was a good candidate for treatment. The emergency department was notified of the infarct before the patient arrived at the hospital, and the fibrinolytic team was notified. When the patient arrived at the emergency department, the fibrinolytic team had been assembled and was waiting. In this scenario, because the team was alerted in advance, the patient received fibrinolytic therapy within 7 minutes of arrival. Although this is only anecdotal evidence and this performance cannot be repeated with every patient, it does serve to illustrate how a team approach (that includes prehospital and hospital personnel) can significantly reduce time to treatment.

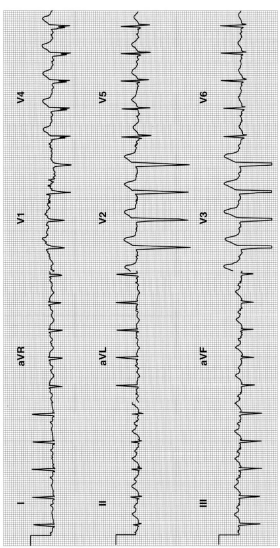

FIGURE **4-9** Prehospital identification of this acute myocardial infarction resulted in a 7-minute door-to-drug time.

Primary percutaneous transluminal coronary angioplasty (PTCA) refers to angioplasty that is performed as a primary reperfusion strategy without prior fibrinolytic therapy. The goal is to achieve reperfusion and salvage of the myocardium. Advantages and disadvantages of primary PTCA versus fibrinolysis in ST-elevation MI are shown in Table 4-2.

TABLE **4-2**	**Primary Percutaneous Transluminal Coronary Angioplasty (PTCA) versus Fibrinolysis in ST-Elevation Myocardial Infarction (STEMI)**
Advantages	**Disadvantages**
Superior vessel patency and flow rates	Lack of generalized availability
Hemodynamic and angiographic data obtained during catheterization can be useful for acute risk stratification	Delay mobilizing cath lab
	Requires skilled interventional cardiologist
Decreased mortality for PTCA compared with fibrinolytic therapy	No large mortality trials
Particularly beneficial in high-risk groups such as older patients, fibrinolytic-ineligible patients, or patients in cardiogenic shock	
Shorter hospital stay	
Improved survival in high-risk patients	
Reduced incidence of reocclusion	
Reduced risk of intracranial hemorrhage	
Reduced rate of recurrent ischemia, reinfarction, stroke, and death	

Adapted from: Fry JA: Acute ST elevation myocardial infarction: primary PTCA in focus on acute coronary syndromes, In Weaver WD, Hudson MP, editors: American College of Cardiology Foundation, 2003.

Primary PTCA

- Recommended as an alternative to fibrinolysis for STEMI if balloon inflation can be performed within 90 ± 30 minutes and in centers with experience and an appropriate laboratory environment
- Preferred for patients younger than 75 years of age with acute MI complicated by cardiogenic shock if the procedure can be performed within 18 hours of the onset of shock
- Should be considered as a reperfusion strategy in candidates for reperfusion who have a contraindication to fibrinolytic therapy

CHAPTER 5

Myocardial Infarction: Recognition and Localization

ECG Changes Due to Infarction

Evolution of a ST-Segment Elevation Myocardial Infarction (STEMI)

The most fundamental use of the ECG is to determine the patient's heart rate and rhythm. When the ECG is used for this purpose, you calculate the number of beats per minute and look closely for the presence of a dysrhythmia. However, different criteria are used to recognize the presence of myocardial infarction (MI).

Although infarction can produce changes in rate and rhythm, infarct recognition on the ECG relies on detecting morphologic changes (i.e., changes in shape) in the QRS complex, T wave, and ST-segment. To review, one of the earliest changes that might be detected is the development of a tall (hyperacute) T wave (Figure 5-1). These T-wave changes may occur within the first few minutes of infarction, during what has been described as the *hyperacute phase* of infarction. These changes are

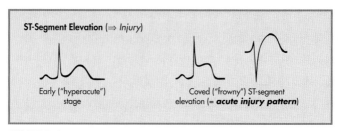

ST-Segment Elevation (⇒ *Injury*)

Early ("hyperacute") stage

Coved ("frowny") ST-segment elevation (= ***acute injury pattern***)

FIGURE **5-1** Hyperacute T waves may be seen in the early stages of infarction.

often not recorded on the ECG because they have typically resolved by the time the patient seeks medical assistance.

Shortly after the hyperacute stage, signs of myocardial injury may develop. ST-segment elevation provides the primary indication of myocardial injury in progress. ST-segment elevation in the shape of a "smiley" face (upward concavity) is usually benign, particularly when it occurs in an otherwise healthy, asymptomatic patient (Figure 5-2, A). The appearance of coved

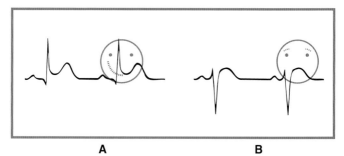

A   B

FIGURE **5-2** **A,** ST-segment elevation in the shape of a "smiley" face (upward concavity) is usually benign, particularly when it occurs in an otherwise healthy, asymptomatic patient. **B,** ST-segment elevation in the shape of a "frowny" face (downward concavity) is more often associated with an acute injury pattern.

("frowny face") ST-segment elevation is called an *acute injury pattern* (Figure 5-2, *B*). Other possible shapes of ST-segment elevation seen with acute MI are shown in Figure 5-3.

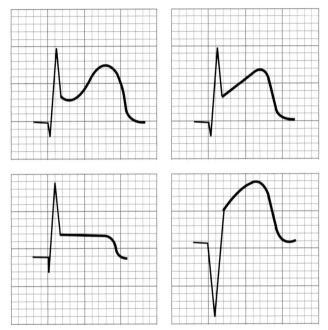

FIGURE **5-3** Variable shapes of ST-segment elevations seen with acute myocardial infarctions.

When looking for ST-segment elevation on a 12-lead ECG, we are particularly interested in the early portion of the ST-segment. Locate the J (junction) point, that is, the connection between the end of the QRS complex and the beginning of the

ST-segment. Locate a QRS complex on the 12-lead ECG, and follow that QRS complex to the end. Look to see where the end of the QRS complex makes a sudden sharp change in direction. That point identifies the J-point.

We should note that there is some difference of opinion as to where ST-segment deviation should be measured. Some authorities simply measure deviation at the J point, whereas others look for deviation 40 ms after the J point. Still others measure ST-segment deviation 60 ms after the J point. Compare the ST-segment deviation to the isoelectric line. The TP segment is best used for this comparison; however, some authorities prefer to use the PR-segment as the baseline.

T-wave inversion, which may occur simultaneously with ST-segment elevation, suggests the presence of ischemia (Figure 5-4). The development of abnormal Q waves provides evidence that tissue death has occurred (Figure 5-5). When combined with ST-segment or T-wave changes, the presence of abnormal Q waves suggests an acute MI (Figure 5-6).

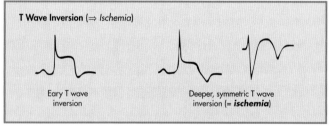

T Wave Inversion (⇒ *Ischemia*)

Eary T wave inversion

Deeper, symmetric T wave inversion (= ***ischemia***)

FIGURE **5-4** T-wave inversion suggests the presence of ischemia.

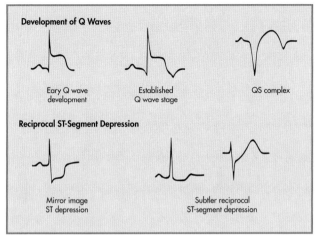

Development of Q Waves

Eary Q wave
development

Established
Q wave stage

QS complex

Reciprocal ST-Segment Depression

Mirror image
ST depression

Subtler reciprocal
ST-segment depression

FIGURE **5-5** The development of abnormal Q waves provides evidence that tissue death has occurred.

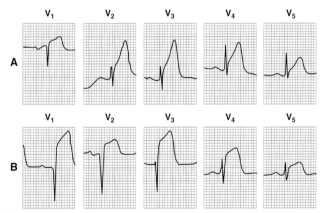

FIGURE **5-6** Chest leads from a patient with an acute anterior wall infarction. **A,** In the earliest phase of the infarction, tall, hyperacute T waves are seen in leads V_2 to V_5. **B,** Several hours later, marked ST-segment elevation is present in the same leads (acute injury pattern), and abnormal Q waves are seen in leads V_1 and V_2.

Contiguous Leads

> *Anatomically contiguous leads* refers to those leads that "see" the same area of the heart.

When ECG changes of MI occur, they are not found in every lead of the ECG. In fact, they are only present in the leads "looking" directly at the infarct site (indicative changes). Indicative changes are significant when they are seen in two anatomically contiguous leads. Two leads are contiguous if they look at the same area of the heart or if they are numerically consecutive *chest* leads (Figure 5-7). Table 5-1 shows the area viewed by each lead of a standard 12-lead ECG.

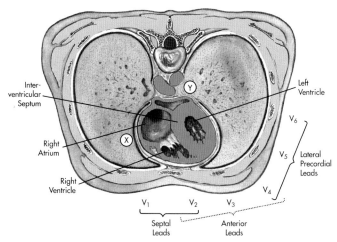

FIGURE **5-7** This is a schematic view of the areas of the heart visualized by the chest leads. Leads V_1, V_2, and V_3 are contiguous. Leads V_3, V_4, and V_5 are contiguous as are as V_4, V_5, and V_6. Note that neither the right ventricular wall (X) nor the posterior wall of the left ventricle (Y) is well visualized by any of the usual six chest leads.

TABLE **5-1**	**Localizing ECG Changes**		
I: lateral	aVR: none	V_1: septum	V_4: anterior
II: inferior	aVL: lateral	V_2: septum	V_5: lateral
III: inferior	aVF: inferior	V_3: anterior	V_6: lateral

Figure 5-8 shows ST-segment elevation of more than 1 mm in leads II, III, and aVF. An inferior wall infarction is suspected to be the cause of the ST-segment elevation. Figure 5-9 shows an ECG with indicative changes in lead I, aVL, and V_2 through V_5. Because these leads view the lateral wall and the anterior wall, an infarction in these areas is suspected.

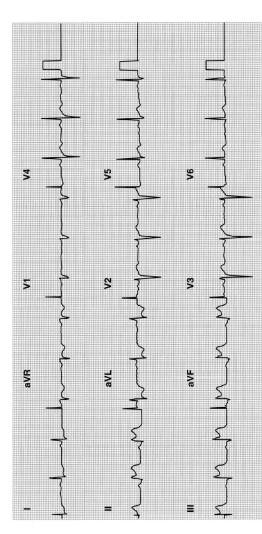

FIGURE 5-8 ST-segment elevation in leads II, III, and aVF reflect an inferior wall injury pattern.

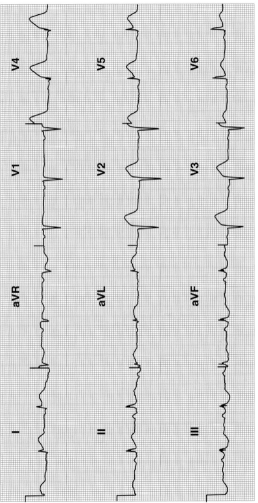

FIGURE **5-9** ST-segment elevation in leads I, aVL, and V₂ through V₅ reflect an anterolateral injury pattern.

Reciprocal Changes

We have said that ECG signs of myocardial injury are reflected by the presence of ST-segment *elevation* in the leads looking directly at the affected area. The uninvolved areas of the heart may show ST-segment *depression.* This is called a *reciprocal* ("mirror image") change. Reciprocal changes are seen in the wall of the heart opposite the location of the infarction (Figure 5-10). Reciprocal changes are usually most readily observed at

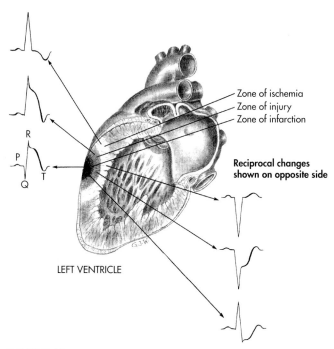

FIGURE **5-10** Zones of ischemia, injury, and infarction showing indicative ECG changes and reciprocal changes corresponding to each zone.

the onset of an infarction and tend to be short lived. When present, reciprocal changes strongly suggest an acute infarction.

Coronary Artery Anatomy

Because MI is the result of an occluded coronary artery, it is worthwhile to develop a familiarity with the arteries that supply the heart. Once the infarction has been recognized and localized, an understanding of coronary artery anatomy makes it possible to predict which coronary artery is occluded.

The main coronary arteries lie on the epicardial surface of the heart and branch into progressively smaller vessels, eventually becoming arterioles and then capillaries. Thus the epicardium has a rich blood supply from which to draw. Branches of the main coronary arteries penetrate into the heart's muscle mass and supply the subendocardium with blood. The diameter of these "feeder branches" is much narrower. The tissue supplied by these "feeder branches" gets enough blood and oxygen to survive, but they do not have much extra.

The heart makes sure to feed itself first because the right and left coronary arteries branch out from the most proximal portion of the aorta. The right coronary artery (RCA) originates from the right side of the aorta and travels along the groove between the right atrium and right ventricle. The marginal branch of the RCA supplies the right atrium and right ventricle.

The left coronary artery (LCA) originates from the left side of the aorta and consists of the left main coronary artery, which divides into two main branches: the left anterior descending (also called the anterior *interventricular*) artery and the left circumflex artery. Branches of the left anterior descending (LAD) artery supply blood to the septum and anterior surfaces of both ventricles. Branches of the LAD include the diagonal and septal arteries. The left circumflex branch supplies blood to the left atrium and the lateral wall of the left ventricle. Branches of the circumflex include the anterolateral and posterolateral marginal arteries.

In about 90% of the population, the RCA forms the posterior descending branch and supplies the inferior wall of the left ventricle. In the remaining 10% of the population, the LCA forms the posterior descending artery. Table 5-2 summarizes the pattern in which coronary arteries most commonly supply the myocardium.

TABLE 5-2	Localization of a Myocardial Infarction (MI)		
Location of MI	Indicative Changes (Leads Facing Affected Area)	Reciprocal Changes (Leads Opposite Affected Area)	Affected Coronary Artery
Anterior	V_3, V_4	V_7, V_8, V_9	Left coronary artery LAD, diagonal branch
Anteroseptal	V_1, V_2, V_3, V_4	V_7, V_8, V_9	Left coronary artery LAD, diagonal branch LAD, septal branch
Anterolateral	I, aVL, V_3, V_4, V_5, V_6	II, III, aVF, V_7, V_8, V_9	Left coronary artery LAD, diagonal branch and/or circumflex branch
Inferior	II, III, aVF	I, aVL	Right coronary artery (most common), posterior descending branch or left coronary artery, circumflex branch
Lateral	I, aVL, V_5, V_6	II, III, aVF	Left coronary artery LAD, diagonal branch or circumflex branch or both
Septum	V_1, V_2	V_7, V_8, V_9	Right coronary artery Left coronary artery LAD, septal branch
Posterior	V_7, V_8, V_9	V_1, V_2, V_3	Right coronary or left circumflex artery
Right Ventricle	V_1R-V_6R	I, aVL	Right coronary artery Proximal branches

LAD, Left anterior descending artery.

Predicting the Site of Coronary Artery Occlusion

With an understanding of coronary anatomy, it is possible to predict which coronary artery is occluded. To identify the site of occlusion, compare the infarct location with the coronary anatomy. If an ECG shows changes in leads II, III, and aVF, suspect an inferior wall infarction. Because the inferior wall of the left ventricle is supplied by the RCA in most of the population, it is reasonable to suppose that this infarct is due to an RCA occlusion. When indicative changes are seen in the leads viewing the septal, anterior, or lateral walls of the left ventricle (V_1-V_6, I, and aVL), it is reasonable to suspect an LCA occlusion.

Assessing the Extent of Infarction

One way to gauge the relative extent or size of an infarction is to evaluate how many leads are showing indicative changes. An ECG showing changes in only a few leads suggests a smaller infarction than one that produces changes in many leads.

Four specific locations along the LCA are identified in Figure 5-11, marked A through D. Consider the tissues that would be affected by an occlusion at each of these sites, and then imagine the leads that might show ECG changes resulting from an occlusion at each site. If an occlusion were to occur at site *A*, then a portion of the anterior wall would be affected, and leads V_3 and V_4 may show indicative changes as a result. If the occlusion were at site *B*, the septum would be affected by the infarction and you would expect to see indicative changes in leads V_1 and V_2 as well. If the circumflex were to occlude at site *C*, you would anticipate a lateral wall infarction with indicative changes shown in leads I, aVL, V_5, and V_6. A more proximal occlusion, such as one at site *D*, would affect a large portion of the left ventricle and could produce indicative ECG changes in most or all of leads I, aVL, and V_1 through V_6.

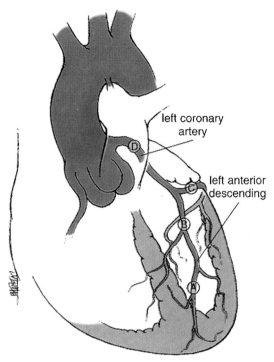

FIGURE **5-11** Extent of infarction as related to various locations of left coronary artery occlusion.

Although the standard 12-lead ECG provides a full view of tissue supplied by the LCA, it gives an incomplete view of tissue supplied by the RCA. In Figure 5-12, three potential sites of an RCA occlusion are marked A through C. An occlusion at site *A* would involve only the distal-most portion of the right coronary artery and would be expected to produce an inferior wall infarction with indicative changes in leads II, III, and aVF. An occlusion at site *B* would involve a larger amount of tissue

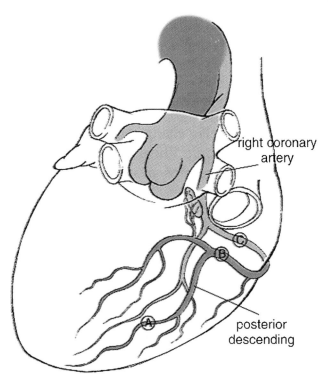

FIGURE **5-12** Extent of infarction as related to various locations of right coronary artery occlusion.

and probably produce a larger infarction. However, there are no leads in the standard 12-lead ECG that "look" at the posterior wall, so indicative changes would only be seen in leads II, III, and aVF. A more proximal occlusion, such as one at site C, would not only involve a much larger portion of the myocardium, but it would also produce an infarction in both ventricles.

Specific Types of Myocardial Infarctions

Anterior Wall

Leads V_3 and V_4 face the anterior wall of the left ventricle. The left main coronary artery supplies the LAD and the circumflex artery. Occlusion of the left main coronary artery (the "widow maker") often leads to cardiogenic shock and death without prompt reperfusion.

Occlusion of the midportion of the LAD results in an anterior infarction (Figure 5-13). However, an infarction involving

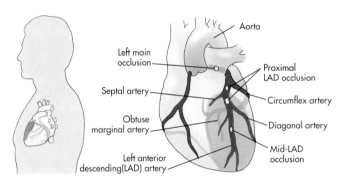

I Lateral	aVR	V_1 Septum	V_4 Anterior
II Lateral	aVL Lateral	V_2 Septum	V_5 Lateral
III Inferior	aVF Inferior	V_3 Anterior	V_6 Lateral

FIGURE **5-13** Anterior wall infarction. Occlusion of the midportion of the left anterior descending *(LAD)* artery results in an anterior infarction. Proximal occlusion of the LAD may become an anteroseptal infarction if the septal branch is involved or an anterolateral infarction if the marginal branch is involved. If the occlusion occurs proximal to both the septal and diagonal branches, an extensive anterior infarction (anteroseptal-lateral myocardial infarction) will result.

the anterior wall is usually not localized only to this area. For example, proximal occlusion of the LAD may become an anteroseptal infarction if the septal branch is involved or an anterolateral infarction if the marginal branch is involved. An example of an infarction involving the anterior wall is shown in Figure 5-14.

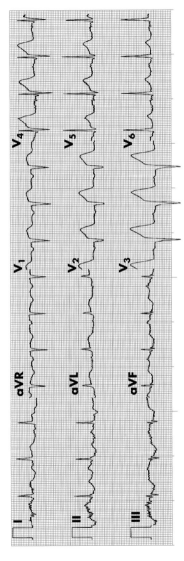

FIGURE 5-14 Extensive anterior infarction.

Inferior Wall

Leads II, III, and aVF view the inferior surface of the left ventricle. In most individuals, the inferior wall of the left ventricle is supplied by the posterior descending branch of the RCA ("right dominant system") (Figure 5-15). Occlusion of the RCA proximal to the marginal branch will result in an inferior wall MI and right ventricular infarction. Occlusion of the RCA distal to the marginal branch will result in an inferior infarction, sparing the right ventricle. Reciprocal changes are observed in leads I and aVL.

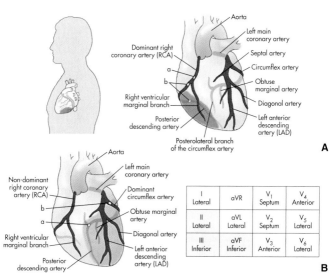

I Lateral	aVR	V₁ Septum	V₄ Anterior
II Lateral	aVL Lateral	V₂ Septum	V₅ Lateral
III Inferior	aVF Inferior	V₃ Anterior	V₆ Lateral

FIGURE **5-15 A,** Inferior wall infarction. Coronary anatomy shows a dominant right coronary artery. Occlusion at point **a** results in an inferior and right ventricular infarction. Occlusion at point **b** is limited to the inferior wall, sparing the right ventricle. **B,** Inferior wall infarction. Coronary anatomy shows a dominant left circumflex artery. Occlusion at point A results in an inferior infarction. An occlusion at B may result in infarction in the lateral and posterior walls.

In some individuals, the circumflex artery supplies the inferior wall through the posterior descending artery ("left dominant system"). Occlusion of the posterior descending artery will result in an inferior infarction; however, a proximal occlusion of the circumflex may result in infarction in the lateral and posterior walls. An example of an infarction involving the inferior wall is shown in Figure 5-16.

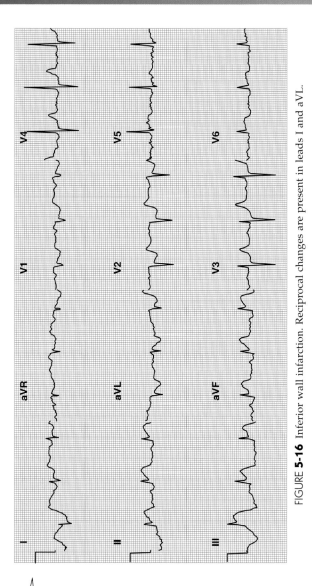

FIGURE **5-16** Inferior wall infarction. Reciprocal changes are present in leads I and aVL.

Lateral Wall

Leads I, aVL, V_5, and V_6 view the lateral wall of the left ventricle. The lateral wall of the left ventricle may be supplied by the left circumflex artery, the left anterior descending artery, or a branch of the RCA (Figure 5-17). An example of an infarction involving the lateral wall is shown in Figure 5-18.

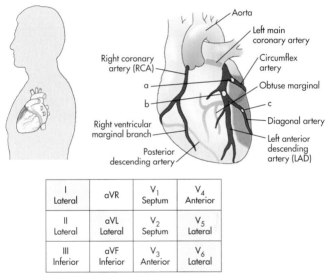

I Lateral	aVR	V_1 Septum	V_4 Anterior
II Lateral	aVL Lateral	V_2 Septum	V_5 Lateral
III Inferior	aVF Inferior	V_3 Anterior	V_6 Lateral

FIGURE **5-17** Lateral wall infarction. Coronary artery anatomy shows occlusion of the circumflex artery **(A)**, occlusion of the proximal left anterior descending artery **(B)**, and occlusion of the diagonal artery **(C)**.

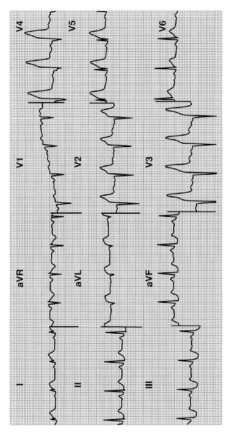

FIGURE **5-18** Acute anterolateral infarction. Note the Q waves in leads aVL, V_2 through V_4, and ST-segment elevation in leads I, aVL, and V_2 through V_5.

Septum

Leads V_1 and V_2 face the septal area of the left ventricle. The septum, which contains the Bundle of His and bundle branches, is normally supplied by the left anterior descending artery (Figure 5-19). If the site of infarction is limited to the septum, ECG changes are seen in V_1 and V_2. If the entire anterior wall is involved, ECG changes will be visible in V_1, V_2, V_3, and V_4. An example of a septal infarction is shown in Figure 5-20.

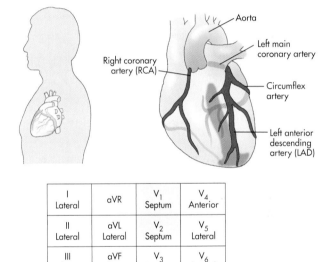

I Lateral	aVR	V_1 Septum	V_4 Anterior
II Lateral	aVL Lateral	V_2 Septum	V_5 Lateral
III Inferior	aVF Inferior	V_3 Anterior	V_6 Lateral

FIGURE **5-19** Septal infarction.

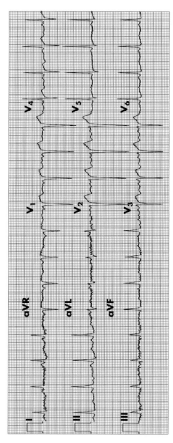

FIGURE **5-20** Septal infarction. Poor R-wave progression.

Posterior Wall

The posterior wall of the left ventricle is supplied by the left circumflex coronary artery in most patients; however, in some patients it is supplied by the RCA (Figure 5-21). Because no leads of a standard 12-lead ECG directly view the posterior wall of the left ventricle, additional chest leads may be used to view the heart's posterior surface. Indicative changes of a posterior wall infarction include ST-segment elevation in these leads.

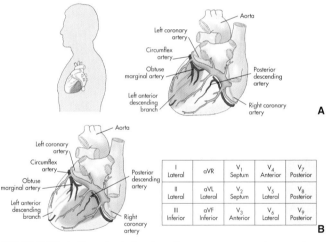

			V₁	V₄	V₇
I Lateral	aVR		V₁ Septum	V₄ Anterior	V₇ Posterior
II Lateral	aVL Lateral		V₂ Septum	V₅ Lateral	V₈ Posterior
III Inferior	aVF Inferior		V₃ Anterior	V₆ Lateral	V₉ Posterior

FIGURE **5-21** **A,** Posterior infarction. Coronary anatomy shows a dominant right coronary artery *(RCA)*. Occlusion of the RCA commonly results in an inferior and posterior infarction. **B,** Coronary anatomy shows a dominant left circumflex artery. Occlusion of a marginal branch is the cause of most isolated posterior infarctions.

If a patient presents with a possible acute coronary syndrome and the only ST-segment change seen on a standard 12-lead ECG is depression (particularly in leads V_1-V_4), strongly consider obtaining posterior chest leads V_7 through V_9 to assess for a possible posterior infarction.

If placement of posterior chest leads is not feasible, changes in the opposite (anterior) wall of the heart can be viewed as reciprocal changes. A posterior wall MI usually produces tall R waves and ST-segment depression in leads V_1, V_2, and to a lesser extent in lead V_3.

Right Ventricular Infarctions

Right ventricular infarction (RVI) should be suspected when ECG changes suggesting an inferior infarction (ST-segment elevation in leads II, III, or aVF) are observed (Figure 5-22). To view

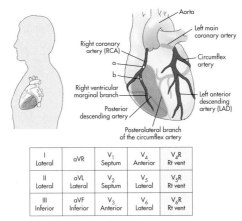

I Lateral	aVR	V_1 Septum	V_4 Anterior	V_4R Rt vent
II Lateral	aVL Lateral	V_2 Septum	V_5 Lateral	V_5R Rt vent
III Inferior	aVF Inferior	V_3 Anterior	V_6 Lateral	V_6R Rt vent

FIGURE **5-22** Right ventricular infarction. Occlusion of the right coronary artery proximal to the right ventricular marginal branch results in an inferior and right ventricular infarction. An occlusion of the right ventricular marginal branch results in an isolated right ventricular infarction.

the right ventricle, right chest leads are used. Placement of right chest leads is identical to placement of the standard chest leads except on the right side of the chest (Figure 5-23). These leads then "look" directly at the right ventricle and can show the ST-segment elevation created by the infarct. If time does not permit the acquisition of all six right-sided chest leads, the lead of choice is V_4R. An example of an infarction involving the right ventricle is shown in Figure 5-24.

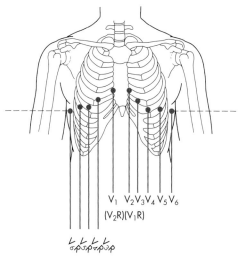

V_1 $V_2V_3V_4$ V_5V_6
$(V_2R)(V_1R)$

FIGURE **5-23** Anatomic placement of the left and right chest leads.

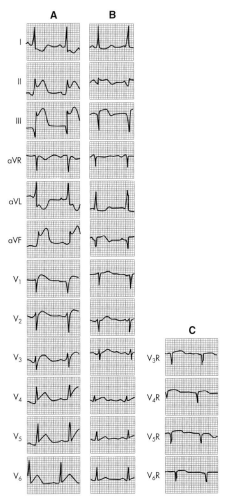

FIGURE **5-24** Evolutionary changes in inferior and right ventricular infarction. **A,** At admission, acute phase. **B,** At 12 hours. **C,** Right chest leads demonstrating right ventricular infarction.

In addition to ECG evidence, certain clinical signs also support the suspicion of RVI. The clinical evidence of RVI involves three components: hypotension, jugular venous distention, and clear breath sounds. Care of the patient with a RVI requires modification of the standard treatment for chest pain.

12-lead ECG Interpretation

We recommend the following approach when reviewing a 12-lead ECG:

1. Assess the quality of the tracing. If baseline wander or artifact is present to any significant degree, note it. If the presence of either of these conditions interferes with the assessment of any lead, use a modifier such as "possible" or "apparent" in your interpretation.
2. Identify the rate and underlying rhythm. Determining rate and rhythm is the first priority when interpreting the ECG. The treatment of life-threatening dysrhythmias initially takes precedence over the acquisition and interpretation of the 12-lead ECG. Yet this does not mean that the 12-lead ECG is of no value when determining rate and rhythm.
3. Examine each lead for the presence of a Q-wave or poor R-wave progression. If a Q wave is present, express the duration in milliseconds. Examine each lead for the presence of ST-segment displacement (elevation or depression). If ST-segment elevation is present, express it in millimeters. Assess the areas of ischemia or injury by assessing lead groupings. Examine the T waves for any changes in orientation, shape, and size. Remember that many infarctions do not produce identifiable changes on the ECG. In addition, certain conditions other than infarction can produce ST-segment elevation. *It is crucial that the ECG is NEVER used to rule out an infarction, especially within the first few hours of symptom onset.* Conversely, conditions other than infarction may be the cause

of ST-segment elevation. Therefore it is important to look for specific evidence of their presence before developing a working diagnosis of infarction.

4. Interpret your findings. Although only a physician can make a final diagnosis of infarction, you must take responsibility for recognizing infarction and take steps to speed the process of data collection, physician evaluation, and, when appropriate, reperfusion therapy. The reduction in time to treatment is your most compelling reason to become familiar with the 12-lead ECG.

CHAPTER 6

Myocardial Infarction: Complications and Treatment

Chest Discomfort

In the setting of an acute coronary syndrome, chest discomfort may be lessened by two primary methods. First, administration of analgesics decreases anxiety and pain, decreases the risk of dysrhythmias, and decreases the catecholamine response, which otherwise could increase the heart's rate, force of contraction, and oxygen demand. Second, vasoactive medications alter the hemodynamics of preload and afterload to reduce the heart's workload and oxygen requirements. For these reasons, a high priority is placed on the relief of cardiac chest discomfort.

Routine measures used in the initial management of the normotensive patient experiencing an acute coronary syndrome include administration of oxygen, aspirin, and nitroglycerin followed by morphine if chest discomfort persists (and there are no contraindications). Right ventricular infarction (RVI) presents an exception to routine measures for chest pain management. In the setting of RVI, the infarction can reduce the output of the right ventricle, with a subsequent reduction in left ventricular filling. Should such a decrease in preload occur, it could potentially decrease left ventricular output as well. This, of course, would result in a decrease in blood pressure.

Morphine and nitroglycerin are vasodilators and thus reduce preload. This reduction in preload, while usually beneficial, can be undesirable in the setting of RVI and may cause profound hypotension. Therefore you must be cautious when administering nitroglycerin and morphine to patients experiencing RVI. If hypotension occurs, it brings with it the serious consequence of a decrease in coronary artery perfusion.

Because the coronary arteries are supplied from the aorta, a decrease in blood pressure will reduce blood flow through the coronary arteries. When this occurs in an already infarcting heart, it can reduce collateral circulation to the infarcting areas or create ischemia in previously unaffected areas of the heart. Therefore hypotension is more than just an inconvenience; it can reduce coronary artery perfusion and worsen the area of injury. Hypotension secondary to pain management is a complication that may be anticipated when treating RVI.

Hypotension Secondary to Right Ventricular Infarction

A common approach to the treatment of hypotension secondary to myocardial infarction (MI, not due to an inappropriate heart rate) has been to administer a small fluid bolus followed by an inotropic drug (a drug that affects cardiac contractility) such as dopamine. RVI is one such underlying factor that should be considered when treating a patient experiencing hypotension in the presence of an inferior wall MI.

When hypotension complicates inferior wall infarction, question whether the hypotension is secondary to a simultaneous RVI. When an inferior wall MI is suspected (indicative changes in leads II, III, and aVF), obtain right-sided chest leads to screen for a RVI. At a minimum, obtain lead V_4R and look for clinical evidence of RVI: jugular venous distention, clear lung sounds, and hypotension. These signs signify the presence of a preload-dependent patient, one who may benefit from fluid therapy. Remember, the problem in this setting is that blood is "stalling" in the right ventricle, resulting in the left ventricle being underfilled. Treatment requires careful fluid administration to raise the left ventricular filling pressure.

If the patient is hypotensive with a known or suspected RVI, repeat intravenous (IV) fluid challenges of 250 to 500 mL (usually with normal saline) may be necessary every 15 minutes, up to 1 to 2 L. The patient's breath sounds and blood pressure must be reassessed after each fluid challenge. If administration of 0.5 to 1.0 L of IV fluid does not improve the patient's blood pressure and cardiac output, a dobutamine infusion is generally used to increase contractility.

It is important to remember that although vigilant fluid administration often resolves the hypotension that accompanies a RVI and improves cardiac output, there also is a simultaneous infarction occurring in the inferior wall of the left ventricle. This coexistent infarction may reduce the left ventricle's pump function and the possibility of provoking pulmonary edema is a very real concern.

Atrioventricular Blocks

The atrioventricular (AV) junction is an area of specialized conduction tissue that provides the electrical links between the atrium and ventricle. If a delay or interruption in impulse conduction occurs within the AV node, bundle of His, or His-Purkinje system, the resulting dysrhythmia is called an *atrioventricular block*. AV block indicates that the electrical impulse originating in the atrium has somehow been blocked from depolarizing the ventricles. AV block can occur at the level of the AV node, at the level of the bundle branches, or at some site in between, such as the bundle of His (Figure 6-1). The two most common sites of AV block are the AV node (nodal block) and the bundle branches (infranodal block) (Table 6-1).

Table **6-1**	Locations of Atrioventricular (AV) Block	
Nodal blocks	AV node	First-degree AV block Second-degree AV block type I Complete (third-degree) AV block
Infranodal blocks	Bundle of His	Second-degree AV block type II (uncommon) Complete (third-degree) AV block
	Bundle branches	Second-degree AV block type II (more common) Complete (third-degree) AV block

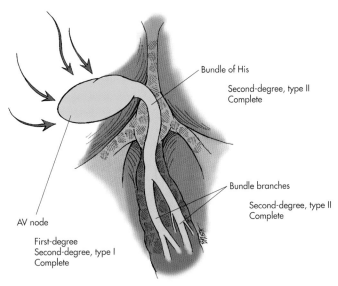

Bundle of His

Second-degree, type II
Complete

Bundle branches

Second-degree, type II
Complete

AV node

First-degree
Second-degree, type I
Complete

FIGURE **6-1** Locations of atrioventricular *(AV)* block.

The AV node's location in the heart is shown in Figure 6-2. The vertical line in the illustration represents the division between the right and the left side of the heart, and the horizontal line represents the division between the atria and the ventricles. The point at which these two lines cross is called the *crux* of the heart—crux means "cross" in Latin—and it is below the crux that the AV node lies. When the coronary anatomy is superimposed over the crux, one can see that the right coronary artery is located nearest to the crux. The right coronary artery supplies the AV node in 90% of the population. Thus, right coronary artery occlusions are associated with AV block occurring in the AV node.

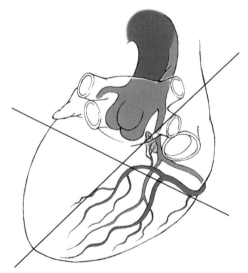

FIGURE **6-2** The right coronary artery is the primary blood supply to the atrioventricular *(AV)* node in about 90% of the population.

The bundle branches are, for the most part, located near the ventricular septum (Figure 6-3). Although some portions of the bundle branches are supplied by the right coronary artery, it is the left coronary artery that supplies most of the bundle branch tissue. Therefore, when AV block occurs in the setting of a left coronary artery occlusion, the location of that AV block is generally in the bundle branches.

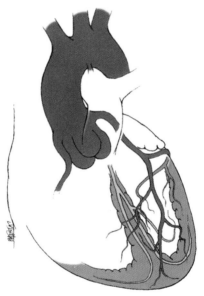

FIGURE **6-3** The left coronary artery supplies most of the bundle branch tissue.

Infarction produces AV block most frequently because of an increase in parasympathetic tone. Local ischemia around the AV node is all that is required to produce AV block. This type of block requires a less severe insult than an AV block caused by serious tissue injury or death. Blocks that are the result of serious tissue injury are usually the result of a more extensive infarction.

First-degree AV block (Figure 6-4) may be a normal finding in individuals with no history of cardiac disease, especially in athletes. First-degree AV block may also occur because of ischemia or injury to the AV node or junction, medications, rheumatic heart disease, hyperkalemia, acute MI (often inferior wall MI), or increased vagal tone. First-degree AV block that occurs with acute MI should be monitored closely.

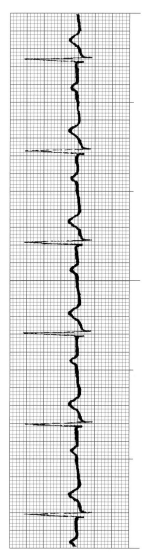

FIGURE **6-4** Sinus rhythm with a first-degree atrioventricular (AV) block.

Second-degree AV block type I (Figure 6-5) is caused by conduction delay within the AV node and is most commonly associated with AV nodal ischemia secondary to occlusion of the right coronary artery. Second-degree AV block type I may also occur because of increased parasympathetic tone or the effects of medications. When associated with an acute inferior wall MI, this rhythm usually occurs because of increased parasympathetic stimulation rather than injury to the conduction system and develops within the first 24 to 48 hours of infarction. This dysrhythmia is usually transient, resolving within 48 to 72 hours as the effects of parasympathetic stimulation disappear.

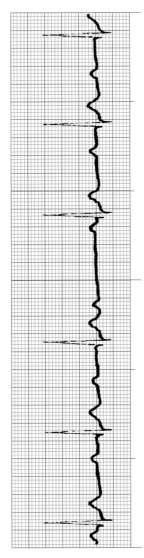

FIGURE **6-5** Second-degree atrioventricular (AV) block type I.

The conduction delay in second-degree AV block type II occurs below the AV node, either at the bundle of His or, more commonly, at the level of the bundle branches (Figure 6-6). The bundle branches receive their primary blood supply from the left coronary artery. Thus disease of the left coronary artery or an anterior MI is usually the cause of this dysrhythmia.

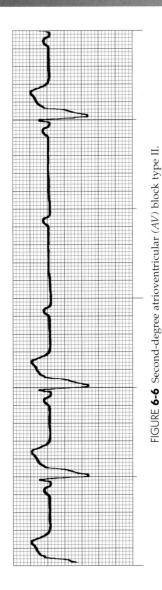

FIGURE **6-6** Second-degree atrioventricular (AV) block type II.

Third-degree AV block associated with an inferior MI is thought to be the result of a block above the bundle of His and often occurs after progression from first-degree AV block or second-degree AV block type I. The resulting rhythm is usually stable, and the escape pacemaker is usually junctional with narrow QRS complexes and a ventricular rate of more than 40 beats/minute (Figure 6-7). Third-degree AV block associated with an anterior MI is usually preceded by second-degree AV block type II or an intraventricular conduction delay (e.g., right or left bundle branch block). The resulting rhythm is usually unstable, and the escape pacemaker is usually ventricular with wide QRS complexes and a ventricular rate of less than 40 beats/minute (Figure 6-8).

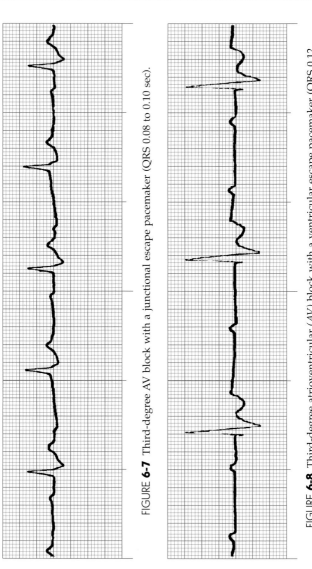

FIGURE **6-7** Third-degree AV block with a junctional escape pacemaker (QRS 0.08 to 0.10 sec).

FIGURE **6-8** Third-degree atrioventricular (AV) block with a ventricular escape pacemaker (QRS 0.12 to 0.14 seconds).

Table 6-2 provides a summary for nodal and infranodal AV blocks.

TABLE 6-2	Nodal and Infranodal Block	
	Nodal Block	**Infranodal Block**
Coronary supply	Right coronary artery	Left coronary artery
QRS width	Usually narrow	Usually wide
Stability	Generally stable	Often unstable
Atropine Response	Usually improves	Often does not respond; may worsen
Infarct Site	Usually inferior or right ventricular	Usually septal or anterior
Cause	Usually increased parasympathetic tone	Usually serious tissue injury
Escape Pacemaker	Junctional, usually reliable	Ventricular, often unreliable

CHAPTER 7

Bundle Branch Block

Structures of the Intraventricular Conduction System

After passing through the atrioventricular node, the electrical impulse enters the bundle of His (also referred to as the *common bundle* or the *atrioventricular bundle*). The bundle of His is normally the only electrical connection between the atria and the ventricles. It is located in the upper portion of the interventricular septum and connects the AV node with the two bundle branches. The bundle of His conducts the electrical impulse to the right and left bundle branches.

The right bundle branch travels down the right side of the interventricular septum to conduct the electrical impulse to the right ventricle. Structurally the right bundle branch is long, thin, and more fragile than the left. Because of its structure, a relatively small lesion in the right bundle branch can result in delays or interruptions in electrical impulse transmission.

The left bundle branch begins as a single structure that is short and thick (the left common bundle branch or main stem) and then divides into three divisions (fascicles) called the *anterior fascicle, posterior fascicle,* and the *septal fascicle.* The anterior fascicle spreads the electrical impulse to the anterior and lateral walls of the left ventricle. This fascicle is thin and vulnerable to disruptions in electrical impulse transmission. The posterior fascicle relays the impulse to the posterior (inferior) portions of the left ventricle, and the septal fascicle relays the impulse to the midseptum (Figure 7-1). The posterior fascicle is short, thick, and rarely disrupted because of its structure and dual blood supply from both the left anterior descending artery and the right coronary artery.

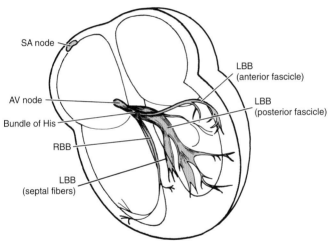

FIGURE **7-1** Conduction system.

During normal ventricular depolarization, the left side of the interventricular septum (stimulated by the left posterior fascicle) is stimulated first. The wave of depolarization then traverses the septum to stimulate the right side. The left and right ventricles are then depolarized simultaneously.

Significance of Bundle Branch Block

In the setting of myocardial infarction (MI), a new onset of bundle branch block (BBB) is a significant finding. Infarct-induced BBB carries with it an increased mortality rate of between 40% and 60%. The rate of cardiogenic shock increases as well, up to 70%. It is not the BBB itself that causes these outcomes. Rather, the new onset BBB indicates extensive infarction, and it is the tissue lost to the infarct that produces the increase in mortality and cardiogenic shock. Because the left anterior descending artery supplies much of the bundle branches, patients experiencing septal and anteroseptal infarctions are most likely to develop BBB.

In the setting of infarction, BBB also identifies patients with a higher likelihood of developing complete AV block. These patients are actually developing a form of infranodal AV block. This is why infranodal AV block often has a wide QRS complex. When BBB is caused by infarct, it can quickly progress to a more complete block with a slow ventricular rate. Another significant aspect of BBB is its ability to mimic the infarct pattern on the ECG. In particular, left BBB (LBBB) can produce ST-segment elevation and wide Q waves that look remarkably similar to infarction.

Causes of Bundle Branch Block

Right BBB (RBBB) can occur in individuals who have no underlying heart disease, but it more commonly occurs in the presence of organic heart disease, with coronary artery disease the most common cause. In patients with acute MI, complete RBBB is present in 3% to 7% of cases. In such cases, it is often accompanied by left anterior hemiblock and is the result of an anterior MI. RBBB occurring as the result of acute MI may require pacemaker intervention. The progression of RBBB to complete AV block occurs twice as often as that of LBBB, especially when RBBB is associated with a fascicular block.

Left BBB may be acute or chronic. Acute LBBB may occur secondary to an anteroseptal (more common) or inferior MI, acute congestive heart failure, acute pericarditis, or myocarditis. Nonischemic diseases, such as Lev's disease and Lenègre's disease, are also capable of producing a BBB. Lev's disease produces BBB through a calcification of the heart's fibrous skeleton. The fibrous skeleton is the infrastructure to which the muscles and valves are attached. Portions of the conduction system are located near the fibrous skeleton or may pass through it. If the fibrous skeleton begins to calcify, part of the electrical conduction system may become "pinched," resulting in a block.

Lenègre's disease is a more diffuse sclerodegenerative disease that tends to affect the distal portions of the conduction system, but it may affect the more proximal portions as well. This process occurs with age, is not related to ischemic heart disease, and is sometimes referred to as the "graying" of the electrical conduction system.

Recognizing Bundle Branch Block

The first rule of BBB recognition is to forget about the notch! Although BBB can put a notch on the QRS complex, it does not always do so, and, when present, the notch is certainly not seen in every lead. Conversely, a notch seen on the QRS complex does not necessitate the presence of a BBB. There is a pervasive association between notching and BBB. People do not easily give up the association, despite its unreliability. Fortunately, there is a simple and reliable method for detecting BBB, the first criteria of which is a widened QRS complex.

When one of the bundles becomes blocked, the impulse that is normally conducted by that bundle branch is interrupted and does not depolarize the intended ventricle. Meanwhile, the other bundle branch is conducting its impulse and depolarizing its respective ventricle. How does the other ventricle depolarize? Very slowly.

For the second ventricle to depolarize, the electrical impulses must trudge through myocardial cells, which are not specialized for electrical conduction. Thus the impulses from one ventricle must be transmitted, cell by cell, to the other ventricle. Because the impulses are wading through the "muck and mire," and not traveling down the "superhighway," ventricular depolarization takes longer to occur. This delay is evidenced in the form of a wide QRS complex. A QRS complex that is 120 ms wide (three small boxes) is a sign of abnormal ventricular conduction. However, BBB is not the only cause of abnormal ventricular conduction; ventricular rhythms are another common cause of wide QRS complexes. Consequently, an additional criterion must also be met to suspect BBB as the cause as opposed to a ventricular rhythm.

Because BBB implies that a supraventricular impulse was aberrantly conducted, and ventricular rhythms are not the result of supraventricular activity, evidence of atrial activity producing the QRS complex rules out the possibility of a ventricular rhythm. Therefore, the second criterion for BBB recognition is evidence of atrial activity producing the QRS complex.

Key Point

Criteria for Bundle Branch Block Recognition

- QRS duration of 120 ms or more (if a complete BBB)
- QRS complexes produced by supraventricular activity (i.e., the QRS complex is not a paced beat, nor did it originate in the ventricles)

There are two important points to remember when examining any ECGs. First, do not trust your eyes. Complexes that are biphasic or triphasic can look narrower than they truly are. Some complexes appear narrow in some leads, but, when measured, are just as wide as the other leads. **Measure the QRS complex duration. Do not trust only your eyes**.

The second point is that the QRS complex may indeed be wider in one lead than it is in another. Variation in QRS duration from lead to lead is often seen and may produce confusion about whether the complex is or is not wide. As a rule, use the widest QRS complex to determine width. Be careful to pinpoint precisely the exact beginning and end of the QRS complex. This can be difficult to do and is sometimes impossible. Therefore **when measuring for bundle branch block, select the widest QRS complex with a discernible beginning and end**.

The criteria for BBB recognition may be found in any lead of the ECG. However, when differentiating RBBB from LBBB, pay particular attention to the QRS morphology in specific leads. Lead V_1 is probably the single best lead to use when differentiating between the two forms of BBB. Before describing the characteristic pattern of each BBB, a review of some basic monitoring principles is required.

> A QRS measuring 100 to 120 ms is called an *incomplete* RBBB or LBBB. A QRS measuring more than 120 ms is called a *complete* RBBB or LBBB. If the QRS is wide but there is no BBB pattern, the term *wide* QRS or intraventricular conduction delay is used to describe the QRS.

Principles of Monitoring

The form of the QRS complex in any given lead is determined by the direction of electrical current in relation to that lead's positive electrode. If an electrical current moves toward the positive electrode, a positive defection is recorded. When current moves away from the positive electrode, a negative deflection is recorded. If the electrical current travels perpendicular to the positive electrode, an equiphasic complex is seen. In an equiphasic complex, the net upward deflection equals the net downward deflection. An equiphasic complex may produce a QRS in which the total upward deflection equals the downward deflection, or it may take the form of an isoelectric line (Figure 7-2).

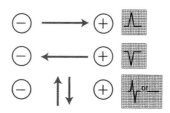

FIGURE **7-2** Basic principles of monitoring.

Differentiating Right from Left Bundle Branch Block

Once the presence of BBB is suspected, an examination of V_1 can reveal whether the block affects the right or the left bundle branch. Following are descriptions of how each type of block affects the direction of electrical current and produces its own, distinct QRS morphology.

Right Bundle Branch Block

The RSR' pattern is sometimes referred to as an "M" or "rabbit ear" pattern.

In RBBB, the electrical impulse travels through the AV node and down the left bundle branch into the interventricular septum. The septum is activated by the left posterior fascicle and is depolarized in a left-to-right direction (event 1 in Figure 7-3). Thus septal depolarization moves in a left-to-right direction,

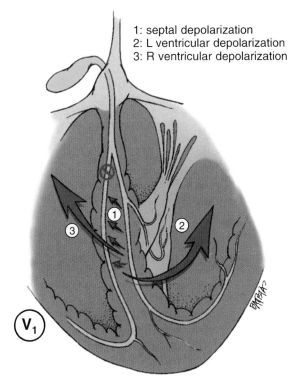

1: septal depolarization
2: L ventricular depolarization
3: R ventricular depolarization

FIGURE **7-3** The RSR' pattern, characteristic of right bundle branch block.

which is toward V_1, and produces an initial small R wave. As the left bundle continues to conduct impulses, the entire left ventricle is depolarized from right to left (event 2). This produces movement away from V_1 and results in a negative deflection (S wave). Now the impulses that depolarized the left ventricle conduct through the myocardial cells and depolarize the right ventricle (event 3). This depolarization creates a movement of electrical activity in the direction of V_1, and so a second positive deflection is recorded (R'). The RSR' pattern is characteristic of RBBB. **Whenever the two criteria for BBB have been met, and V_1 displays an RSR' pattern, RBBB is suspected**.

Left Bundle Branch Block

In LBBB, the septum is depolarized by the right bundle branch, as is the right ventricle. The septum is part of the left ventricle and, thus, the wave of myocardial depolarization has begun with the net movement of current going away from V_1 (event 1 in Figure 7-4). This movement of current continues to move away from V_1 as the rest of the left ventricle is depolarized (event 2), and the QRS complex continues in its negative direction. Thus LBBB produces a QS pattern in V_1. **When BBB is known to exist and a QS pattern is seen in V_1, LBBB is suspected**.

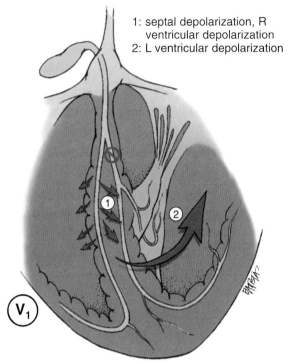

1: septal depolarization, R
    ventricular depolarization
2: L ventricular depolarization

FIGURE **7-4** A QS pattern in V_1, characteristic of left bundle branch block.

An Easier Way

Unfortunately, not every bundle branch block presents with a clear RSR' or QS pattern in V_1. Often, the pattern more closely resembles a qR pattern or an rS pattern (Figure 7-5), making the differentiation less clear.

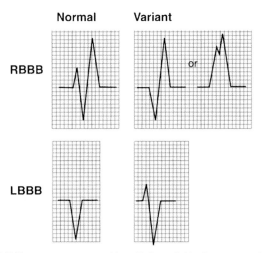

FIGURE **7-5** Variant patterns of bundle branch block as seen in lead V_1.

The final portion of the QRS complex is referred to as the *terminal force.* To identify the terminal force, first locate the J-point. From the J-point, move backward into the QRS and determine whether the last electrical activity produced an upward or downward deflection. An example of the terminal force in both RBBB and LBBB is illustrated in Figure 7-6. If the right bundle branch is blocked, then the right ventricle will be depolarized last and the current will be moving from the left ventricle to the right. This will create a positive deflection in the terminal force of the QRS complex in V_1. If the left bundle branch is blocked, the left ventricle will be depolarized last, and the current will flow from right to left. This will produce a negative deflection in the terminal force of the QRS complex seen in V_1.

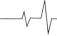

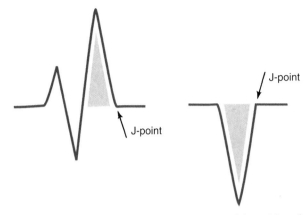

FIGURE **7-6** Determining the direction of the terminal force. Move from the J-point into the QRS complex and determine whether the terminal portion (last 0.04 seconds) of the QRS complex is a positive (upright) or negative (downward) deflation. If the two criteria for bundle branch block *(BBB)* are met and the terminal portion of the QRS is positive, right BBB is most likely present. If the terminal portion of the QRS is negative, left BBB is most likely present.

Therefore, to differentiate RBBB from LBBB, look at V_1 and determine whether the terminal force of the QRS complex is directed upward or downward. If it is directed upward, an RBBB is present (the current is moving toward the right ventricle and toward V_1). An LBBB is present when the terminal force of the QRS complex is directed downward (the current is moving away from V_1 and toward the left ventricle). This rule is especially helpful when RSR′ and QS variants are present (see Figure 7-5).

A simple way to remember this rule has been suggested by Mike Taigman and Syd Canan and is demonstrated in Figure 7-7. They recognized the similarity between this rule and the turn indicator on a car. When a right turn is made, the turn indicator is lifted up. Likewise, when an RBBB is present, the terminal force of the QRS complex points up. Conversely, left turns and LBBB are directed downward.

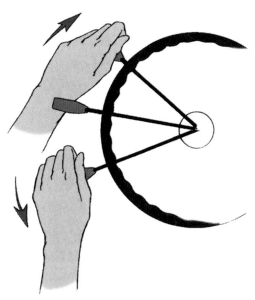

FIGURE **7-7** Differentiating between right and left bundle branch block. The *turn signal theory:* right is up; left is down.

Acute Coronary Syndromes Imitators

ST-Segment Elevation

ST-segment elevation is not caused by myocardial infarction (MI) per se. The theories are complex, but ST-segment elevation is caused by changes that affect ventricular repolarization or ventricular depolarization or both. MI produces ST-segment elevation because the infarction affects ventricular repolarization or depolarization. Likewise, any condition that affects ventricular repolarization or depolarization can also produce ST-segment elevation.

Numerous conditions can cause ST-segment elevation. Hypothermia, increased intracranial pressure, electrolyte imbalance, and medications are just a few of these conditions.

A Common Feature of LBBB, LVA, and Ventricular Beats

Awareness of the particular feature shared by left bundle branch block (LBBB), left ventricular hypertrophy (LVH), and ventricular beats is helpful before progressing to the specific criteria for each. The common feature relates to an ECG pattern in which the QRS complex and the T wave are oppositely directed. In other words, when the QRS complex points down, the T wave points up and vice versa.

This phenomenon would hardly be noteworthy in a discussion of infarction except for one important fact: The T wave often "drags" the ST-segment along with it. Thus, when the QRS complex is primarily negative, the T wave will be positively deflected, and it can drag the ST-segment up with it. This is how LBBB, LVH, and ventricular rhythms can masquerade as an infarction. Figure 8-1 demonstrates this pattern. Note how the T wave "drags" the ST-segment along with it. This phenomenon produces ST-segment elevation in leads with a negatively deflected QRS complex. Additionally, the negative deflection may produce a Q wave or QS complex equal to or more than 40 ms in duration. This further clouds the interpretation by giving the appearance of pathologic Q waves.

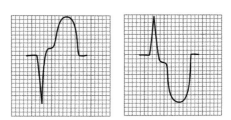

FIGURE **8-1** When left bundle branch block, ventricular rhythms, and left ventricular hypertrophy *(LVH)* are present, the T wave is opposite in direction from the QRS complex. Note how the ST-segment is shifted in the direction of the T wave.

Left Bundle Branch Block

ECG Recognition

Essentially two conditions must exist to suspect bundle branch block. First, the QRS complex must have an abnormal duration (120 ms or more in width); second, the QRS complex must arise as the result of supraventricular activity (this excludes ventricular beats). If these two conditions are met, delayed ventricular conduction is assumed to be present, and bundle branch block is the most common cause of this abnormal conduction.

Once a bundle branch block has been detected, lead V_1 may be used to differentiate right from LBBB. In lead V_1, determine the direction of the terminal (last) force of the QRS complex. If the terminal force points up, suspect a right bundle branch block (RBBB). If the terminal force points down, suspect am LBBB.

When BBB is present, ST-segment elevation is often seen in leads with negatively deflected QRS complexes. This situation occurs most frequently in the presence of LBBB and is generally seen in leads V_1, V_2, and V_3 but sometimes extends to V_4 and beyond. Figure 8-2 demonstrates this pattern.

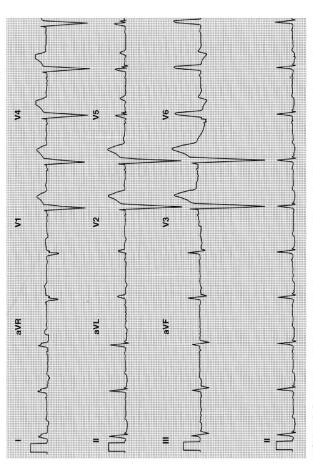

FIGURE **8-2** Left bundle branch block is present. Note the ST-segment elevation in the leads with negatively deflected QRS complexes.

Right bundle branch block rarely produces ST-segment elevation because most of the leads remain positively deflected. Occasionally, when the inferior leads (II, III, and aVF) happen to be negatively deflected, a RBBB may produce ST-segment elevation in those leads and may occasionally mimic an inferior wall infarction. Although this combination is possible, LBBB is by far the more common cause of ST-segment elevation.

Ventricular Rhythms

Impulses originating in the ventricles may be the result of either natural pacemaker sites or of implanted pacemakers. As with BBB, ventricular rhythms may exhibit ST-segment elevation that is not due to any infarct-related causes. This imitation ST-segment elevation is seen when the QRS complex is negatively deflected.

Ventricular Paced Rhythm

In many ways, a ventricular paced beat is a man-made LBBB. Consider that when LBBB occurs, the electrical impulse travels down the right bundle branch, depolarizes the right ventricle, and spreads through the myocardium to depolarize the left ventricle. Pacemakers are most often introduced into the right ventricle attached to the right ventricular wall. When a pacemaker fires, it sends its impulse into the right ventricle, which depolarizes, and the impulse is spread through the myocardium to depolarize the left ventricle. The similarity between the two is shown in Figure 8-3.

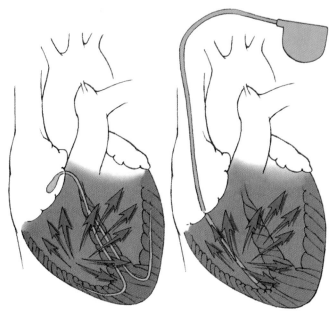

FIGURE **8-3** The patterns of left bundle branch block and a ventricular pacemaker are similar because in both cases the ventricular impulse begins in the right ventricle and conducts throughout the myocardium to depolarize the left ventricle.

Similarly, spontaneous impulses originating in the ventricles can produce ST-segment elevation, which is often seen accompanying a negatively deflected premature ventricular complex (PVC). If a ventricular rhythm is present, the ECG may show ST-segment elevation in the leads that are negatively deflected (Figure 8-4).

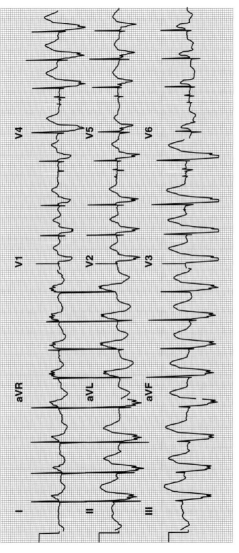

FIGURE **8-4** An example of a ventricular rhythm producing ST-segment elevation.

Left Ventricular Hypertrophy

Left ventricular hypertrophy is an enlargement of the left ventricle. The enlargement results from a prolonged state of overfilling in the left ventricle or from its pumping against increased resistance. The ECG does not detect every case of LVH, but there are clues that, when present, strongly favor its presence.

Whereas BBB increases the *width* of the QRS complex, LVH increases the *amplitude* because of the increase in electrical activity. To detect evidence of LVH on the ECG, use the following method.

Step 1
- Compare V_1 and V_2 and determine which lead has the deepest S wave.
- Determine the depth of the deeper S wave in millimeters (count the small boxes; one box equals 1 mm).

Step 2
- Compare V_5 and V_6 and determine which lead has the tallest R wave.
- Determine the height of the taller R wave in millimeters (count the small boxes).

Step 3
- Add the height of the taller R wave and the deeper S wave.
- If the number is equal to or greater than 35, suspect LVH. Use the example in Figure 8-5 to practice this method.

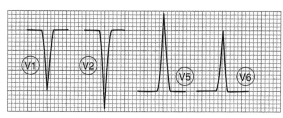

FIGURE **8-5** *Step 1*, In comparing V_1 and V_2, the S wave is greater in V_2 and equals about 19 mm in depth. *Step 2*, The R wave in V_5 is taller than in V_6. The height of the R wave equals 19 mm. *Step 3*, The sum of the depth of the S wave plus the height of the R wave is 19 + 19 = 38. Voltage criteria for LVH have been met.

The ECG shown in Figure 8-6 meets the voltage criteria for LVH. Note that the ST-segment is elevated in leads V_1, V_2, and V_3. Also note the ST-segment depression shown in leads V_5 and V_6. This conforms to the pattern described earlier in which negatively deflected QRS complexes display ST-segment elevation whereas positively deflected QRS complexes show ST-segment depression.

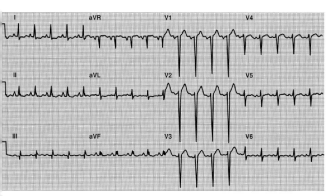

FIGURE **8-6** ST-segment elevation noted in the presence of left ventricular hypertrophy.

Pericarditis

Pericarditis can produce a number of changes in the ECG. ST-segment elevation occurs frequently and may be noted in any lead. Because the ST-segment elevation is related to diffuse patches of inflammation around the pericardium, and not due to an occluded coronary artery, ST-segment elevation is usually diffuse and not strictly grouped into leads that are anatomically contiguous. Pericarditis can also produce PR-segment depression. When the ST-segment is compared with a depressed PR-segment, it can give the appearance of ST-segment elevation. Using both the TP segment and the PR-segment to establish the isoelectric line will minimize this illusion.

Another change that pericarditis may bring to the ECG is a notching of the J-point. Although not exclusive to pericarditis, J-point notching signifies the possibility of a noninfarct cause of ST-segment elevation. Figure 8-7 illustrates how some leads show examples of true ST-segment elevation, and other leads appear elevated as the result of PR-segment depression, and a few display J-point notching.

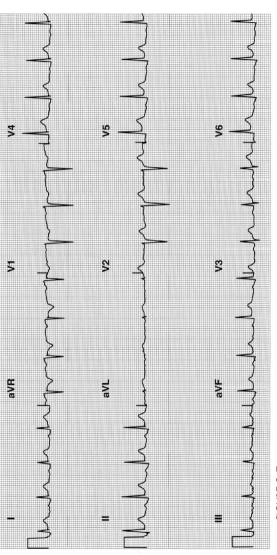

FIGURE **8-7** The pattern of pericarditis. Note the diffuse pattern of ST-segment elevation, PR-segment depression in lead II, and J-point notching in leads II, V5, and V6.

The recognizable ECG features of pericarditis are subtle and can easily be overlooked or misinterpreted. Therefore it is often the clinical presentation of pericarditis that is first recognized. Once pericarditis is suspected, the ECG can be closely examined (or reexamined) for substantiating evidence. Table 8-1 compares the ECG and clinical features of MI and pericarditis.

TABLE **8-1**	Clinical Presentation of Acute Myocardial Infarction and Pericarditis	
	Myocardial Infarction	**Pericarditis**
Chest pain (nature)	Pressure	Stabbing
Chest pain (radiation)	Left arm, shoulder, jaw	Base of neck, trapezius area
Chest pain (aggravation)	Unaffected by movement	Affected by movement, respiration, swallowing, etc. May improve when leaning forward
ST-segment elevation	Appears in anatomically contiguous leads	Diffuse across ECG
PR-segment depression	Uncommon	Common, may give appearance of ST-segment elevation

Early Repolarization

Early repolarization produces an infarct-like pattern on the ECGs of healthy, asymptomatic patients. Early repolarization is considered a normal variant and does not indicate any underlying pathology.

Early repolarization produces ST-segment elevation that is most often seen in the chest leads. Additionally, early repolarization produces tall T waves resembling those seen in the hyperacute phase of MI. This combination creates a pattern on the ECG that closely resembles that of anterior or anterolateral infarction.

J-point elevation in early repolarization is usually accompanied by a slur, oscillation, or notch at the end of the QRS just before and including the J-point. As with pericarditis, a notch at the J-point causes one to consider noninfarct conditions as possible explanations for the ST-segment elevation. In general, R-wave and T-wave voltages are large in early repolarization.

The pattern of early repolarization is shown in Figure 8-8. Table 8-2 presents an overview of five conditions and how they mimic infarction.

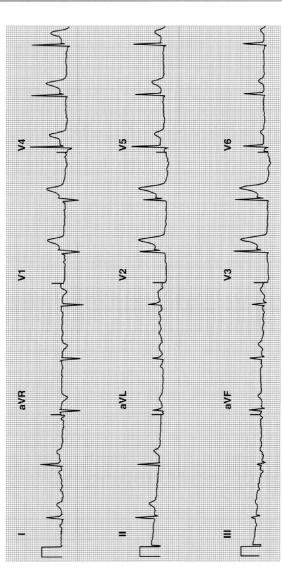

FIGURE **8-8** An example of ST-segment elevation resulting from early repolarization.

TABLE 8-2	Overview of the Acute Coronary Syndrome Imitators	
Condition	Infarction Resemblance	Recognition
Left bundle branch block	ST-segment elevation in the negatively deflected leads, usually V_1-V_3	QRS Complex ≥ 120 ms
	QS complexes in the negatively deflected leads, usually V_1-V_3	QRS complex produced by supraventricular activity
		QS complex, or negative terminal force in V_1
Ventricular rhythms	ST-segment elevation in the negatively deflected leads	Wide QRS complex following pacer spikes (if noticeable)
	QS complexes in the negatively deflected leads	Negative terminal force in V_1 (right ventricle paced)
Left ventricular hypertrophy	ST-segment elevation in the negatively deflected leads, usually V_1-V_3	Choose deepest S wave from V_1 and V_2
		Choose tallest R wave from V_5 and V_6
		Add deflections of tallest R wave and deepest S wave
		Suspect LVH if total ≥ 35
Pericarditis	Elevates ST-segments in multiple leads	ST-segment elevation not in anatomical grouping
		PR-segment depression
		Notching of the J-point
Early repolarization	ST-segment elevation, particularly in anterior or anterolateral leads	Notching of the J-point
	Tall T waves	Patient may be asymptomatic
		Most common in athletic African-American men < 40 yr of age

References

1. Alpert JS, Thygesen K, et al: Myocardial infarction redefined—a consensus document of The Joint European Society of Cardiology/American College of Cardiology Committee for the redefinition of myocardial infarction. *J Am Coll Cardiol* 36(3):959-969, 2000.
2. Ryan TJ, Antman EM, Brooks NH, et al: 1999 update: ACC/AHA guidelines for the management of patients with acute myocardial infarction: a report of the American College of Cardiology/American heart Association Task Force on Practice Guidelines (Committee on Management of Acute Myocardial Infarction). *J Am Coll Cardiol* 1999;34:890-911. Available at http://www.acc.org/clinical/guidelines.
3. Ohman EM, Armstrong PW, Christenson RH, et al: Cardiac troponin T levels for risk stratification in acute myocardial ischemia. GUSTO IIA Investigators, *N Engl J Med* 335:1333-1341, 1996.

Illustration Credits

FIGURE 1-1 Thibodeau G, Patton K: *Structure and function of the body,* ed 12, St. Louis, 2004, Mosby.

FIGURE 1-2 Herlihy B, Maebius N: *The human body in health and illness,* ed 2, St. Louis, 2003, WB Saunders.

FIGURE 1-3 Herlihy B, Maebius N: *The human body in health and illness,* ed 2, St. Louis, 2003, WB Saunders.

FIGURE 1-4 Herlihy B, Maebius N: *The human body in health and illness,* ed 2, St. Louis, 2003, WB Saunders.

FIGURE 2-2 Thelan L, Urden L, Lough M et al: *Critical care nursing: diagnosis and management,* ed 3, St. Louis, 1998, Mosby.

FIGURE 2-4 Clochesy J, Breu C, Cardin S, et al: *Critical care nursing,* ed 2, Philadelphia, 1996, WB Saunders.

FIGURE 2-6 Thelan L, Urden L, Lough M et al: *Critical care nursing: diagnosis and management,* ed 3, St. Louis, 1998, Mosby.

FIGURE 2-7 Aehlert B: *ECGs made easy,* ed 2, St. Louis, 2002, Mosby

FIGURE 2-10 Conover M: *Understanding electrocardiography,* ed 8, St. Louis, 2003, Mosby.

FIGURE 2-11 Thibodeau G, Patton K: *Anatomy and physiology,* ed 5, St. Louis, 2003, Mosby

FIGURE 2-12 Thibodeau G, Patton K: *Anatomy and physiology,* ed 5, St. Louis, 2003, Mosby.

FIGURE 2-13 Surawicz B, Knilans T: *Chou's electrocardiography in clinical practice: adult and pediatric,* ed 5, Philadelphia, 2001, WB Saunders.

FIGURE 3-2 Clochesy J, Breu C, Cardin S et al: *Critical care nursing,* ed 2, Philadelphia, 1996, WB Saunders.

FIGURE 3-3 Lounsbury P, Frye S: *Cardiac rhythm disorders,* ed 2, St. Louis, 1992, Mosby.

FIGURE 4-1 Braunwald E, Goldman L: *Primary cardiology,* Philadelphia, 1998, WB Saunders.

FIGURE 4-2 Falk E, Anderson HR: Pathology of atherosclerotic plaque: stable, unstable, and infarctional. In Rougin G, Califf R, O'Neill R, et al, editors: *Interventional cardiovascular medicine: principles and practice,* New York, 1994, Churchill Livingstone.

FIGURE 4-3 Braunwald E, Goldman L: *Primary cardiology,* Philadelphia, 1998, WB Saunders.

FIGURE 4-4 Thelan L, Urden L, Lough M et al: *Critical care nursing: diagnosis and management,* ed 3, St. Louis, 1998, Mosby.

FIGURE 4-5 Thibodeau G, Patton K: *Anatomy and physiology,* ed 5, St. Louis, 2003, Mosby

FIGURE 4-6 Thelan L, Urden L, Lough M et al: *Critical care nursing: diagnosis and management,* ed 3, St. Louis, 1998, Mosby.

FIGURE 4-8 Mosby: *Managing major diseases: cardiac diseases,* St. Louis, 1998, Mosby.

FIGURE 5-1 Grauer K: *A practical guide to ECG interpretation,* ed 2, St. Louis, 1998, Mosby.

FIGURE 5-2 Grauer K: *A practical guide to ECG interpretation,* ed 2, St. Louis, 1998, Mosby.

FIGURE 5-3 Goldberger A: *Clinical electrocardiography: a simplified approach,* ed 6, St. Louis, 1999, Mosby.

FIGURE 5-4 Grauer K: *A practical guide to ECG interpretation,* ed 2, St. Louis, 1998, Mosby.

FIGURE 5-5 Grauer K: *A practical guide to ECG interpretation,* ed 2, St. Louis, 1998, Mosby.

FIGURE 5-6 Goldberger A: *Clinical electrocardiography: a simplified approach,* ed 6, St. Louis, 1999, Mosby.

FIGURE 5-7 Grauer K: *A practical guide to ECG interpretation,* ed 2, St. Louis, 1998, Mosby.

FIGURE 5-8 Johnson R, Swartz M: *A simplified approach to electrocardiography,* Philadelphia, 1986, WB Saunders.

FIGURE 5-9 Hampton J: *The ECG Made Easy,* ed 6, London, 2003, Churchill Livingstone.

FIGURE 5-10 Thelan L, Urden L, Lough M et al: *Critical care*

nursing: diagnosis and management, ed 3, St. Louis, 1998, Mosby.

FIGURE 5-18 Hampton J: *The ECG in practice,* ed 4, London, 2003, Churchill Livingstone.

FIGURE 5-24 Kinney M: *Andreoli's comprehensive cardiac care,* ed 8, St. Louis, 1995, Mosby.

FIGURE 6-1 Aehlert B: *ECGs Made Easy,* ed 2, St. Louis, 2002, Mosby

FIGURE 6-4 Aehlert B: *ECGs Made Easy,* ed 2, St. Louis, 2002, Mosby.

FIGURE 6-5 Aehlert B: *ECGs made easy,* ed 2, St. Louis, 2002, Mosby.

FIGURE 6-6 Aehlert B: *ECGs made easy,* ed 2, St. Louis, 2002, Mosby.

FIGURE 6-7 Aehlert B: *ECGs made easy,* ed 2, St. Louis, 2002, Mosby.

FIGURE 6-8 Aehlert B: *ECGs made easy,* ed 2, St. Louis, 2002, Mosby.

FIGURE 7-1 Thelan L, Urden L, Lough M et al: *Critical care nursing: diagnosis and management,* ed 3, St. Louis, 1998, Mosby.

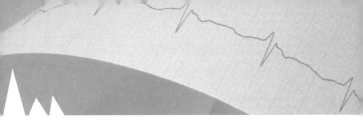

Subject Index

Page numbers followed by *f* indicate figures; page numbers followed by *t* indicate tables.

A

Accuracy, in 12-lead ECG
    acquisition, 37-44, 38t,
      39f-43f
    calibration, 43, 43f
    frequency response, 41-42,
      42f
    lead placement, 37-41, 38t,
      39f-41f
    paper speed, 44
ACSs. *See* Acute coronary
    syndromes (ACSs)
Acute coronary syndromes
    (ACSs), 49-70. *See also specific*
    disorder
    angina, 57-59, 58f
    assessment of, initial, 65-66
    coronary artery obstruction,
      50-53, 51f-53f
    imitators of, 131-143, 132f,
      134f, 136f, 137f, 139f, 141f,
      142t, 144f, 145t
    infarction, 54-70
    injuries, 54-70

Acute coronary syndromes
    (ACSs) (*Continued*)
    interventions for, 67-69, 68f,
      69t
    ischemia, 54-70
    management of, immediate,
      goals in, 49
    MI, 59-65, 60f, 64f
Acute injury pattern, 72f, 73
Angina, 57-59, 58f
    described, 57
    discomfort due to, sites for, 57,
      58f
    stable, 58
    unstable, 59
Anterior fascicle, 118, 119f
Anterior interventricular artery, 8
Anterior wall MI, 87-88, 87f, 89f
Arteriosclerosis, 50
Artery(ies). *See specific artery, e.g.,*
    Left coronary artery
Artifact(s), 36
    in 12-lead ECG acquisition, 46
Atherosclerosis, 50

Atria, 2
Atrioventricular (AV) blocks
   first-degree, 109, 110f
   infranodal, 117, 117t
   locations of, 106, 106f, 106t
   MI and, 105-117, 106f-108f,
      106t, 110f, 112f, 114f, 116f,
      117t
   nodal, 117, 117t
   second-degree
      type I, 111, 112f
      type II, 16, 17f
   third-degree, 115, 116f
Atrioventricular (AV) bundle, 118
Atrioventricular (AV) node, 106f,
   106t, 107, 107f
AV blocks. See Atrioventricular
   (AV) blocks
Axis determination, two-lead
   method of, 35, 35t
Axis deviation, 32-35, 34f, 35t

B
Baseline, 23
BBB. See Bundle branch block
   (BBB)
Blood flow, through heart, 4-6,
   5f, 7f
Bundle branch(es)
   divisions of, 118-119, 119f
   of heart, 106, 106f, 106t, 108,
      108f
Bundle branch block (BBB),
   118-130
   causes of, 120-121
   left, 121, 126, 127f, 133-135, 134f
      ECG recognition in, 133-135,
         134f
      features of, 131-132, 132f,
         145t
      vs. right, 124-126, 125f, 127f

Bundle branch block (BBB)
      (Continued)
   monitoring of, principles of,
      123-124, 124f
   patterns of, 128f
   recognition of, 121-123
   right, 120-121, 124-126, 125f,
      135
      vs. left, 124-126, 125f, 127f
   significance of, 120
Bundle of His, 12, 105, 106, 106f,
   106t, 118

C
Cable(s), in 12-lead ECG
   acquisition, problems
   associated with, 46, 47
CAD. See Coronary artery
   disease (CAD)
Calibration, in 12-lead ECG
   acquisition, 43, 43f
Cardiac. See also Heart
Cardiac action potential, 10
Cardiac cells, types of, 9-10, 10t
Cardiac output, 9
Cell(s). See Pacemaker cells; specific
   types, e.g., Cardiac cells
Chest discomfort, MI and,
   103-104
Chest leads, placement of, 19-20,
   19f, 20f
Circulation, coronary, 6-9, 7f.
   See also Coronary
   circulation
Clarity, in 12-lead ECG
   acquisition, 36-37
Common bundle, 118
Complex(es), 27-31, 28f, 29f, 31f,
   32f
Conduction system, 11-13, 11f,
   119, 119f

Contiguous leads, 30
  in MI, 76-77, 76f, 77t, 78f, 79f
Coronary artery(ies)
  anatomy of, 81-82, 83t
  left, 108, 108f
    in coronary circulation, 8
  right, in coronary circulation,
    8
Coronary artery disease (CAD),
  53
Coronary artery obstruction,
  50-53, 51f-53f
Coronary artery occlusion, site
  of, prediction of, 84
Coronary circulation, 6-9, 7f
  anterior view of, 55, 55f
  components of, 6
  coronary veins in, 9
  left coronary artery in, 8
  right coronary artery in, 8
Coronary sinus, 9
Coronary veins, in coronary
  circulation, 9
Crux, of heart, 107

D

Depolarization, 10-11
Depression, ST-segment, 80
Diabetes mellitus, MI in, 62
Diagnostic quality, 42

E

Early repolarization, 142-143,
  144f, 145t
ECG. See Electrocardiogram
  (ECG)
Einthoven's equilateral triangle,
  33, 34f
Electrocardiogram (ECG)
  described, 14
  electrodes in, 14

Electrocardiogram (ECG)
    (Continued)
  examination of, point to
    remember in, 123
  function of, 14
  in left BBB, 133-135, 134f
  in MI, 62-65, 64f, 71-81, 72f-76f,
    77t, 78f-80f
  reciprocal changes due to, in
    MI, 80-81, 80f
  12-lead. See 12-lead ECG
Electrocardiogram (ECG) paper,
  25-27, 25f, 26f
  speed of, 44
  time as factor in, 25, 25f
  voltage in, 26
Electrode(s), 14
  in 12-lead ECG acquisition,
    problems associated with,
    46
Electromagnetic interference, in
  12-lead ECG acquisition, 48
Emergency Medical Services
  (EMS), 47
EMS. See Emergency Medical
  Services (EMS)
Endocardium, 3, 54, 54f
Epicardium, 3, 54, 54f
Diabetes mellitus, MI in, 62
Extensive anterior MI, 88, 89f
Extreme right axis deviation,
  35

F

Face(s)
  "frowny," 72-73, 72f
  "smiley," 72-73, 72f
Fascicle(s), of bundle branch, 118,
  119f
Fiber(s), Purkinje, 13
Fibrinolysis, PTCA vs., in MI, 69,
  69t

Frequency response, in 12-lead ECG acquisition, 41-42, 42f
"Frowny" face, 72-73, 72f

H

Heart. *See also under* Cardiac
    blood flow through, 4-6, 5f, 7f
    bundle branches of, 106, 106f, 106t, 108, 108f
    chambers of, 2
    conduction system of, 11-13, 11f
    layers of, 3
    location of, 1-2, 1f
    as pump, 9
    valves of, 3-4, 4t
His-Purkinje system, 105
Hyperacute phase of infarction, 71-72, 72f
Hypotension, secondary to right ventricular infarction, MI and, 104-105

I

Indeterminate deviation, 35
Infarction(s)
    myocardial. *See* Myocardial infarction (MI)
    right ventricular, hypotension secondary to, MI and, 104-105
    of ventricular wall, locations of, 54, 54f
    zones of, 80f
Inferior wall MI, 90-91, 90f, 92f
Infranodal AV blocks, 117, 117t
Injury(ies), zones of, 80f
Interatrial septum, 2
Interval(s), 27-31, 28f, 29f, 31f, 32f
Interventricular artery, anterior, 8

Interventricular septum, 2
Intraventricular conduction system, structures of, 118-120, 119f
Ischemia, 50
    myocardial, 56, 56t
    zones of, 80f
Isoelectric line, 23

J

J-point, 29, 29f, 74, 143
Junctional escape pacemaker, third-degree AV block with, 115, 116f

L

Lateral wall MI, 93, 93f, 94f
Lead(s)
    axis deviation in, 32-35, 34f, 35t
    chest, placement of, 19-20, 19f, 20f
    contiguous, 30
        in MI, 76-77, 76f, 77t, 78f, 79f
    limb, 17-18, 18f
    placement of, 15-20, 15t, 16f, 18f-20f
        chest leads, 19-20, 19f, 20f
        described, 15, 15t, 16f
        limb leads, 17-18, 18f
    in 12-lead ECG acquisition, 37-41, 38t, 39f-41f
    what is "seen" by, 21-23, 21t, 22f, 24f
Left anterior descending (LAD) artery, 8, 81
Left axis deviation, 35
Left circumflex (LCx) artery, 8
Left coronary artery, 108, 108f
    in coronary circulation, 8
Left main coronary artery, 8

Left ventricular hypertrophy
(LVH), 138-139, 139f, 145t
features of, 131-132, 132f,
145t
Limb leads, placement of, 17-18,
18f
LVH. *See* Left ventricular
hypertrophy (LVH)

M

Mean axis, 33
MI. *See* Myocardial infarction
(MI)
Monitor quality, 42
Myocardial cells, 9-10, 10t
Myocardial infarction (MI),
59-65, 60f, 64f, 71-102
anterior wall, 87-88, 87f, 89f
atypical presentation of,
61-62
AV blocks and, 105-117,
106f-108f, 106t, 110f, 112f,
114f, 116f, 117t
causes of, 57
chest discomfort with, 103-104
clinical presentation of, 61
complications of, 103-117
contiguous leads in, 76-77, 76f,
77t, 78f, 79f
coronary artery anatomy,
81-82, 83t
coronary artery occlusion in,
site of, prediction of, 84
defined, 59
described, 59-60
in diabetics, 62
diagnosis of, 60, 60f
ECG changes due to, 62-65,
64f, 71-81, 72f-76f, 77t,
78f-80f

Myocardial infarction (MI)
(*Continued*)
extensive anterior, 88, 89f
extent of, assessment of,
84-101, 85f-87f, 89f,
90f, 92f-96f, 99f,
101f-100f
hyperacute phase of, 63, 64f,
71-72, 72f
hypotension secondary to right
ventricular infarction
with, 104-105
inferior wall, 90-91, 90f, 92f
lateral wall, 93, 93f, 94f
localization of, 71-81, 72f-76f,
77t, 78f-80f, 82, 83t
non-ST-segment elevation in,
53
posterior wall, 97-98, 99f
recognition of, 71-81, 72f-76f,
77t, 78f-80f
right ventricular, 98-101,
101f-100f
of septum, 95, 95f, 96f
ST-segment elevation in, 53,
71-75, 72f-75f
PTCA *vs.* fibrinolysis in, 69,
69t
reciprocal changes in, 80-81,
80f
symptoms of, 61-62
treatment of, 103-117
12-lead ECG interpretation of,
101-102
types of, 87-98, 87f, 89f, 90f,
92f-96f, 99f
Myocardial injury, 56-57
Myocardial ischemia, causes of,
56, 56t
Myocardium, 3, 54

N

Negative degrees, 34
"No man's land," 35
Nodal AV blocks, 117, 117t
Node(s), AV, 106f, 106t, 107,
    107f
Non-ST-segment elevation MI
    (NSTEMI), 53, 62
Northwest deviation, 35
NSTEMI. *See* Non-ST-segment
    elevation MI (NSTEMI)

P

Pacemaker(s)
    junctional escape, third-degree
        AV block with, 115, 116f
    ventricular escape, third-
        degree AV block with, 115,
        116f
Pacemaker cells, 10, 10t
Paper, ECG, 25-27, 25f, 26f, 44.
    See also Electrocardiogram
    (ECG) paper
Pericarditis, 140-142, 141f, 142t,
    145t
    ECG features of, 142, 142t
    pattern of, 141f
Pericardium, 3
Plaque(s)
    stable, 50, 51f
    vulnerable, 51, 51f-53f
Positive degrees, 34
Posterior fascicle, 118, 119f
Posterior wall MI, 97-98, 99f
Primary percutaneous
    transluminal coronary
    angioplasty (PTCA)
    fibrinolysis *vs.*, in STEMI, 69,
        69t
    primary, 70

PTCA. *See* Primary percutaneous
    transluminal coronary
    angioplasty (PTCA)
Purkinje fibers, 13

Q

Q wave, 27-28, 28f, 73-74, 75f, 132
QRS complex, 27-30, 28f, 29f,
    31f, 32f, 73-74, 128, 130, 132,
    132f, 133, 134f, 139, 139f
QS complex, 132
QS pattern, 126, 127f, 129
QT interval, 30, 32f
Quality
    diagnostic, 42
    monitor, 42

R

R wave, 27-28, 138, 139f
Reciprocal change, 80, 80f
Repolarization, 10-11
    early, 142-143, 144f, 145t
Right axis deviation, 34-35
Right coronary artery, in
    coronary circulation, 8
Right ventricular infarctions,
    hypotension secondary to,
    MI and, 104-105
Right ventricular MI, 98-101,
    101f-100f
RSR' pattern, 125f, 126, 127, 129

S

S wave, 27-29, 138, 139f
Segment(s), 27-31, 28f, 29f, 31f,
    32f
Septal fascicle, 118, 119f
Septum
    interventricular, 2
    MI of, 95, 95f, 96f

Sinus(es), coronary, 9
Sinus rhythm, with first-degree AV block, 109, 110f
"Smiley" face, 72-73, 72f
Speed, in 12-lead ECG acquisition, 44
Stable angina, 58
Stable plaques, 50, 51f
ST-elevation MI (STEMI), 53
STEMI. *See* ST-elevation MI (STEMI)
ST-segment depression, 80
ST-segment elevation, 136, 137f, 139, 144f
  causes of, 131
ST-segment elevation in MI (STEMI), 29-30, 32f
  evolution of, 71-75, 72f-75f
  PTCA *vs.* fibrinolysis in, 69, 69t
Subendocardial area, 3, 54, 54f
Subepicardial area, 3, 54, 54f

T

T wave, 29-31, 31f, 132, 132f
Terminal force, 128, 129, 129f
Time, in ECG paper, 25, 25f
Troubleshooting, in 12-lead ECG acquisition, 46-48, 47f
"Turn signal theory," 130, 130f
T-wave inversion, 74, 74f-75f
12-lead ECG
  acquisition of, 36-48
    artifacts, 46
    electromagnetic interference and, 48
    equipment-related problems in, 46
    goals in, 36-44, 38t, 39f-43f
      accuracy, 37-44, 38t, 39f-43f

12-lead ECG (*Continued*)
  acquisition of (*Continued*)
    goals in (*Continued*)
      clarity, 36-37
      speed, 44
    patient movement-related problems in, 46-48, 47f
    process of, 44, 45f
    technique-related problems in, 46-48, 47f
    troubleshooting in, 46-48, 47f
  electrodes in, 14
  format of, 26-27, 26f
  introduction to, 14-35
  lead placement in, 15-20, 15t, 16f, 18f-20f. *See also* Lead(s), placement of
  in MI, interpretation of, 101-102
  paper for, 25-27, 25f, 26f

U

Unstable angina, 59

V

Valve(s), heart, 3-4, 4t
Vein(s), coronary, in coronary circulation, 9
Ventricle(s), 2
Ventricular beats, features of, 131-132, 132f, 145t
Ventricular escape pacemaker, third-degree AV block with, 115, 116f
Ventricular paced rhythms, 135-136, 136f, 137f, 145t
Ventricular rhythms, 135-136, 136f, 137f, 145t
  ventricular paced rhythms, 135-136, 136f, 137f, 145t

Ventricular wall, infarctions of, locations of, 54, 54f
Voltage, in ECG paper, 26
Vulnerable plaques, 51, 51f-53f

W
Wave(s). *See specific types, e.g.,* Q wave
Waveform(s), 27-31, 28f, 29f, 31f, 32f